Adverse Outcomes in Maternity Care

Proceeds from the sales of *Adverse Outcomes in Maternity Care* will be donated to **Baby Lifeline**. This charity is dedicated to providing care for unborn and newborn babies, and their mothers.

For Books for Midwives:

Commissioning Editor: Mary Seager
Development Editor: Catharine Steers
Project Controller: Morven Dean
Designer: George Ajayi

Adverse Outcomes in Maternity Care

Implications for Practice, Applying the Recommendations of the Confidential Enquiries

Edited by

Grace Edwards RN RM ADM Cert. Ed M, Ed PhD

Consultant Midwife in Public Health, Liverpool Women's Hospital, Crown Street, Liverpool

Foreword by

Michael Weindling BSc MA MD FRCP FRCPCH

Professor of Perinatal Medicine, University of Liverpool
Chairman, CEMACH

BfM Books *for* Midwives

EDINBURGH LONDON NEW YORK OXFORD PHILADELPHIA ST LOUIS SYDNEY TORONTO 2004

BOOKS FOR MIDWIVES
An imprint of Elsevier Limited

First published 2004

ISBN 0 7506 8789 4

British Library Cataloguing in Publication Data
A catalogue record for this book is available from the British Library

Library of Congress Cataloging in Publication Data
A catalog record for this book is available from the Library of Congress

The
publisher's
policy is to use
**paper manufactured
from sustainable forests**

Printed in China

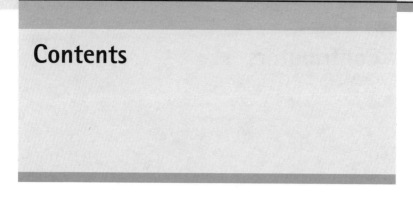

Contents

Contributors

Ruth Bell
Clinical Lecturer in Public Health Medicine, School of Population and Health Sciences (Epidemiology and Public Health), Faculty of Medical Sciences, University of Newcastle, Newcastle upon Tyne

Judith Bush
Senior Research Associate, School of Population and Health Sciences (Epidemiology and Public Health), Faculty of Medical Sciences, University of Newcastle, Newcastle upon Tyne

Jean Chapple MBChB MCommH FFPHM FRCP DRCOC DCH
Consultant in Obstetric and Perinatal Epidemiology, Westminster Primary Care Trust, London and Honorary Senior Lecturer, Department of Epidemiology and Public Health, Imperial College, London

Richard Congdon MA(Oxon) ACA
Chief Executive CEMACH, Confidential Enquiry into Maternal and Child Health, Baker Street, London

Tricia Cresswell
Director of Public Health, Durham and Chester le Street PCT, John Snow House, University of Durham Science Park, Durham

Grace Edwards RN RM ADM Cert. Ed M Ed Phd
Consultant Midwife in Public Health, Liverpool Women's Hospital, Crown Street, Liverpool

Peter Fleming
Professor of Infant Health, Division of Child Health, University of Bristol, UBHT Education Centre, Bristol

Jason Gardosi MD FRCOG FRCSED
Professor of Maternal and Perinatal Health, University of Warwick; Director, West Midlands Perinatal Institute, Crystal Court, Aston Cross, Birmingham

Melanie J. Gompels RN RM BA(Hons) MSc
CEMACH Regional Manager, South East and the Channel Islands Wessex Institute for Health and Research Development, University of Southampton, Southampton

Gwyneth Lewis MBBS MSc MRCPG FFPMH FRCOG
Director, UK Confidential Enquiries into Maternal Deaths, Wellington House, London

Alison Miller RN RM AdvDip(Mid)
Programme Director CEMACH, Confidential Enquiry into Maternal and Child Health, Baker Street, London

Judith Rankin
Senior Research Associate, School of Population and Health Sciences (Epidemiology and Public Health), Faculty of Medical Sciences, University of Newcastle, Newcastle upon Tyne

Marjorie Renwick
Regional Manager CEMACH, Operational Manager, Regional Maternity Survey Office, Royal Victoria Infirmary, Newcastle upon Tyne

Mary Sidebotham
Consultant Midwife, Stepping Maternity Hospital, Stockport, Cheshire

Rosie Thompson
Regional Coordinator for the South Western Region, Division of Child Health, University of Bristol, UBHT Education Centre, Bristol

Martin Ward Platt MD FRCPCH
Consultant Neonatologist, Clinical Director, Northern Regional Maternity Survey Office, Royal Victoria Infirmary, Newcastle upon Tyne

Foreword

This book will be of the greatest interest to all concerned with the care of pregnant women and their babies. The authors are all experts in their fields and closely involved with the Confidential Enquiry into Maternal Deaths (CEMD) and the Confidential Enquiry into Stillbirths and Deaths in Infancy (CESDI). Their writings are authoritative and summarize clearly the major findings of these two confidential enquiries.

CEMD was established in 1952 and has produced reports every 3 years. Gwyneth Lewis has been involved with the organization for many years. She sets out the global picture, reminding us that in developed countries one woman in 5000 will die of pregnancy-related complications, compared with one in 11 in developing countries. Even in the UK, where thromboembolism is the leading cause of death, there is no room for complacency: the maternal mortality rate is highest among the women of low socio-economic class, very young girls and certain ethnic groups. Furthermore, care was substandard in 50% of direct deaths. It is also timely to note that many mothers who died in the most recent triennium were overweight: obesity was a factor in nearly half (46%) of cases of uterine rupture and 11% of shoulder dystocia.

Jean Chapple, an epidemiologist, gives an historical perspective. She reminds us that because of confidential enquiries, practitioners cannot bury their mistakes without learning from them. These lessons have been passed on to colleagues and there have been improvements. In 1928, 3000 mothers and 41 000 babies died in England and Wales: the maternal mortality rate was 4.4 deaths per 1000 maternities and the perinatal mortality rate was 60.8 per 1000 total births. Compare this with the 1990s when there were only about 40 maternal deaths a year and the perinatal mortality rate was about 8 per 1000 births.

Antepartum stillbirths and antenatal care are considered by Jason Gardosi, who is Director of the West Midlands Perinatal Institute. He reminds us that panel assessments often found that there was a failure to monitor fetal growth or to act appropriately when there was a problem, a theme that is picked up later by Alison Miller.

Mary Sidebotham considers the impact of the confidential enquiry programme on intrapartum deaths. She highlights failures due to lack of senior involvement, failures of communication, poor record keeping, ineffective monitoring of fetal well-being during labour and lack of resources. There were failures of neonatal resuscitation too: lack of organization and inappropriate responses. Mary calls for better training and improved resources, which could remedy many of these problems. The Royal Colleges are now fully committed to the principals of lifelong learning and continuing professional development and it seems that her plea is at last being heard.

CESDI was established in 1992 by the Department of Health to reduce death in late fetal life and infancy by identifying where suboptimal care might have contributed to a poor outcome. It produced reports annually. Alison Miller is a midwife, formerly a regional manager CESDI and now a director of CEMACH. She considers the outcome of premature births from a midwifery perspective. In its Project 27/28, CESDI used a number of original methodologies, including the Delphi technique to define national standards and a case-control approach, with enquiry panel members being unaware of the outcome at the start of the enquiry. The study defined several characteristics of mothers that were associated with an increased risk of preterm birth: smoking, ethnic background with language barriers, and multiple pregnancy. Antenatal steroids and postnatal surfactant have made an enormous difference to the outcome of this vulnerable group, but there were still deficiencies in fetal well-being assessments among the babies who died. As in other areas Alison emphasises the importance of adequate training in all aspects of neonatal management.

Rare adverse events are considered by Melanie Gompels and Grace Edwards. They start by reminding us that the enquiries have been able to highlight aspects of care that traditional scientific studies may miss. Their chapter focuses on midwifery aspects of suboptimal care. Planned home birth has been shown to have good outcomes for mothers and babies but the confidential enquiries still found that there were cases of delay in calling or support after the start of labour and communication issues. Prediction of shoulder dystocia is difficult, but traditional clinical skills remain important and three-quarters of cases are successfully delivered by a combination of traction and McRoberts's manoeuvre.

Rosie Thompson and Peter Fleming give a fascinating account of the background to the studies that led to the dramatic and very welcome reduction in the incidence of sudden unexplained deaths in infancy. The respective roles of various professionals are considered including those of health visitors and social workers.

The authors of the penultimate chapter recognize that confidential enquiry panels have an important educational role for participants. They argue strongly that confidential enquiries, when run in the CESDI fashion, can be a powerful tool both to educate and to drive change through the experiences of participants on the panels. One of the benefits of panel participation is the development of inter-professional respect and to do this in a non-hierarchical setting where the quest for the truth is a team effort.

The CEMD and CESDI have just been transformed into a new organization, the confidential enquiry into Maternal and Child Health (CEMACH). This book is particularly welcome because it is being published when CEMACH is just one year old. Its chief executive is Richard Congdon, who summarizes the vision for CEMACH in the final chapter. CEMACH is committed to the case control approach and its studies will be scientifically robust. Ownership of CEMACH by the professions is seen as vitally important. CEMACH's mission is to continue the work of CEMD and CESDI and extend it into childhood: it aims to improve health care and the outcomes for mothers, babies and children by continuing national confidential enquiries, and by disseminating the findings and recommendations as widely as possible.

Liverpool, UK   Michael Weindling
                                                     February 2004

Acknowledgements

I would like to thank CEMACH for their support in producing this book, in particular Richard Congdon, the Chief Executive of CEMACH for reviewing the manuscript and offering advice on editing. I would also like to thank Michael Weindling, the chair of CEMACH for providing the foreword to this book.

I'm indebted to the support from Elsevier, in particular Catharine Steers who has given me invaluable support throughout my first editorial journey.

I would also like to thank Judy Ledger and the staff of Baby Lifeline, the charity who will benefit from the royalties of this book, for their total confidence in my ability as a first time editor. I hope I have fulfilled that confidence.

Thanks must also go to the contributors to this book, who have helped to ensure that my first editorial undertaking was an interesting one!

Finally I would like to dedicate this book to my family, particularly Robin my husband, Katrina my daughter, my mum Grace and my sister Angie, who follow my professional progress with pride.

The authors would like to thank the Earl and Countess of Wessex Charitable Trust who donated the funds for this project.

Chapter 1

An introduction to maternal, perinatal and infant mortality

Jean Chapple

Physicians are of all men the most happy; what good success soever they have, the world proclaimeth, and what faults they commit the earth covereth.
(Francis Quarles 1592–1644)

As part of high-quality clinical care, the public and patients want up-to-date information and their own views and preferences considered – but most of all, they want good outcomes of care. Maternity care in the UK has always been ahead of other services in trying to work in partnership with women and their families, and has also led the way in looking at outcomes of care for both the mother and her baby. Confidential enquiries ensure that general practitioners, obstetricians, midwives, anaesthetists, paediatricians, neonatal nurses and pathologists cannot bury their mistakes without learning from them and passing on those lessons to colleagues. More recent enquiries have also looked at the contribution of social conditions to maternal and infant death, with messages for public health specialists, local authorities, social services, the police and politicians.[1]

This chapter looks at the history of the study of deaths of mothers and babies, how information about deaths is defined, collected and analyzed, and the development of confidential enquiries.

COLLECTING INFORMATION ON THE DEATHS OF MOTHERS AND BABIES

One of the earliest outcome measures used in the NHS was perinatal mortality. This measure was first proposed in an article published in 1948,[2] that suggested combining stillbirth and first-week death rates, as the time trends for early neonatal deaths were more like those for stillbirths than other death rates in infancy (see Tables 1.1 and 1.2). If we are to use mortality rates to study outcomes of pregnancy, then how can we collect these figures so that they are accurate?

A walk around any churchyard will confirm the short life expectancy of previous generations. Families depended on their children to support them in an age when there were no state benefits. So many children died young that Victorian families had on average eight children to try to ensure that at least two survived to adulthood to support their parents and family. However, childbirth was unsafe for mothers. Two hundred years later, parents in developing countries face the same dilemma – they need children to support them, but repeated childbirth leads to the risk of the mother dying herself. High birth and death rates in rural communities led to slow overall population growth. The UK was the first country to industrialize in the early 19th century. The move of agricultural workers from the country to towns in order to work in factories led to great changes in lifestyle. Acts passed to provide education for children and stop child labour meant that children were no longer early wage earners, but needed investment and support from their family until their education was over. Better living conditions, food supply and sanitation led to fewer deaths from infectious disease. Life expectancy increased and the UK underwent the first demographic transition, led by a decline in death rates whilst the birth rate remained the same, causing population growth, although there was no change in fertility patterns. As children became more dependent, there was a decline in birth rate, and population growth became more stable. However, the age breakdown of the population had changed dramatically, with a much older population and a smaller proportion of children.

Table 1.1   Definitions

WHO definitions of maternal mortality

A **maternal death** is the death of a woman while pregnant or within 42 days of termination of pregnancy, irrespective of the duration and the site of the pregnancy, from any cause related to or aggravated by the pregnancy or its management, but not from accidental or incidental causes.

A **late maternal death** is the death of a woman from direct or indirect obstetric causes more than 42 days, but less than 1 year after termination of pregnancy.

A **pregnancy-related death** is the death of a woman while pregnant or within 42 days of termination of pregnancy, irrespective of cause of death.

Maternal deaths should be subdivided into two groups accordingly:
Direct obstetric deaths are those resulting from obstetric complications of the pregnant state (pregnancy, labour and puerperium), from interventions, omissions, incorrect treatment or from a chain of events resulting from any of the above.

Indirect obstetric deaths are those resulting from previous existing disease or disease that developed during pregnancy and which was not due to direct obstetric causes, but which was aggravated by physiological effects of pregnancy. (*Source:* International statistical classification of disease and health related problems, tenth revision, 1992.)

Definitions of live and still birth, and perinatal death

A **liveborn baby** is a child who breathes or shows signs of life after complete expulsion from its mother, regardless of length of gestation.

A **stillbirth** is defined in England and Wales as a child issuing forth from its mother after the 24th completed week of pregnancy which did not at any time after being completely expelled from its mother breathe or show any other signs of life. (Section 41 of the Births and Deaths Registration Act 1953, amended 1 October 1991.)

A **perinatal death** is a fetal death after 24 completed weeks gestation and before 6 completed days of life.

Governments need to know population numbers to plan taxation and public services such as schools and hospitals. The UK government started taking censuses in 1801, and a census has been held every 10 years since, with the exception of 1941. These provide a 'snapshot' of the population, but governments need information on who enters that snapshot by birth or immigration and who leaves it by death or emigration. Industrialization altered methods of collecting information about populations as well as populations themselves. With the move from the country to towns and cities, authorities could no longer rely on information from parish baptismal and burial records. In 1837, a law was passed to make it a statutory requirement to register all

Table 1.2 Definitions of mortality rates

The **maternal mortality rate** – the number of maternal deaths per 100 000 maternities (all pregnancies, including miscarriages, abortions and ectopic pregnancies).

The **perinatal mortality rate (PNMR)** per thousand births is calculated from:

$$\frac{\text{(Stillbirths + deaths at 0-6 days after live birth)}}{\text{Live births + stillbirths}} \times 1000$$

and is the number of stillbirths and early neonatal deaths (those occurring in the first week of life) per 1000 total births (live and stillbirths).

Stillbirth rate – the number of stillbirths per 1000 total births (live births and stillbirths).

Neonatal death rate – the number of neonatal deaths (occurring within the first 28 days of life) per 1000 live births.

Early neonatal death rate – the number of early neonatal deaths (occurring within the first 7 days of life) per 1000 live births.

Infant mortality rate – deaths under the age of 1 year following a live birth, per 1000 live births.

births and deaths in the locality in England and Wales where the birth or death had taken place. Registration became statutory in Scotland in 1855.[3] For deaths related to pregnancies, the number of deaths (the numerator data) is divided by the total number of births or pregnancies (denominator data) to give mortality rates.

BIRTH REGISTRATION

Parents are required to give details of the baby and demographic data, such as their own date and place of birth, to the registrar within 42 days of the birth. Certain details, such as parity of the mother and the occupation of the father (to determine social class) are requested only for legitimate babies. As over one-third of babies are now born to parents who are not married, this information is not obtained for an increasingly large proportion of births.

Important information, such as birthweight, gestational age and ethnic group of parents, is completely omitted from initial collection of registration data.

All liveborn babies must be registered. A liveborn baby is a child who breathes or shows signs of life after complete expulsion from its mother, regardless of length of gestation. This categorization varies from one country to another, as there are different legal definitions excluding live births below defined lower limits of gestational age or birthweight. Laws relating to the timing of registration may also affect whether the child is certified as live or stillborn.[4]

Stillbirths and neonatal deaths must all be registered. The certificates made out by the registrar include the medical cause of death, certified by the doctor in attendance. Stillbirth certificates act as both a birth and death certificate, and the child's name can be included, as well as the birthweight, gestational age and cause of death, which may be certified by a midwife. Since 1986, a neonatal certificate has been issued that, like a stillbirth certificate, collects data on maternal causes contributing to the death for babies who die before the 28th day of life.

This current definition of stillbirth came into force on 1 October 1992; prior to this, the cut off gestational age was 28 weeks. This change in definition has increased the perinatal mortality rate (PNMR), as babies dying between 25 and 28 weeks are now included in the figures, although the Office of National Statistics (ONS) continues to supply figures based on both definitions. Stillborn babies are defined by the time after which they were born, rather than the gestation at which they died, so a papyraceous twin who has died months before its sibling is born should be registered as a stillbirth.

Individual judgement may also play a part in certification of perinatal deaths[5] and judgements about viability.[6] Some fetuses are born so early that they are not viable but may still show visible signs of life for a few minutes. The current abortion law in England, Wales and Scotland allows termination of pregnancy for severe fetal malformation at any gestational age. If the termination is carried out after 24 weeks' gestation and the fetus is dead at birth, it should officially be registered as a stillbirth, and the legal forms relating to termination of pregnancy must also be completed. If feticide is not carried out prior to delivery, such a fetus may be live born and die after delivery, and this should again be registered as a live birth and subsequent death, with official disposal of the body, and with completed termination documentation. However, it is not unknown for clinicians to be influenced by perceptions of how the parents will feel about official form filling and by financial considerations for the parents with regard to maternity benefit and the cost of burial. This is understandable – the legal cut-off points are artificial and parental grief pays no regard as to what stage in pregnancy a baby is lost – but, technically, illegal. Place of delivery of premature babies of less than 24 weeks' gestation (on the delivery suite or on a gynaecology ward) may affect classification and hence figures for perinatal mortality.[5] The onus of judgement regarding viability and classification is often placed on relatively junior staff. There is a theoretical possibility that there may be pressure on clinical staff to regard a fetus as non-registrable if the clinical performance of their unit is judged on its crude PNMR alone.

NOTIFICATION OF BIRTHS

An increasing interest in improving maternal and child health at the beginning of the 20th century led to the introduction of another system of collecting data about births within hours rather than the 6 weeks allowed by law for birth registration. This ensures that midwives, health visitors and doctors are aware that a baby has been born and can offer clinical support and advice. The attendant at the birth has to notify the designated medical officer (usually the Director of Public Health) of the local health authority of any birth occurring in that authority, in writing, within 36 hours of birth. This system gives the opportunity to collect information on birthweight, which since 1978 has been statutorily transferred from the notification system to the birth registration system to provide national statistics on birthweight. Birth attendants are also asked to notify ONS about congenital malformations noted within 10 days of birth to give a national picture of the birth prevalence of malformations. This requirement started in 1964 in response to the thalidomide tragedy.

MEASURING MATERNAL DEATHS

Measurement of maternal mortality is more complex than measurement of the deaths of babies because of difficulties in collecting denominator data. There is no law requiring registration or notification of pregnancies that do not result in birth or in termination at any stage. We can only estimate the number of miscarriages and ectopic pregnancies each year. The death of any woman has to be registered and since 1927 death certificates have asked for 'factors contributing to the death but not related to the immediate cause', which should include pregnancy. It is difficult to assess how many deaths from illegal abortion were registered properly prior to the Abortion Act of 1967.

DEVELOPMENT OF CONFIDENTIAL ENQUIRIES

A sixteen year old unmarried primigravida from Social Class V has an antepartum haemorrhage at 28 weeks' gestation followed by spontaneous labour and the premature delivery of an infant who rapidly develops respiratory distress syndrome and dies on the second postnatal day. The post mortem examination demonstrates hyaline membrane disease and intraventricular haemorrhage ...

The paediatricians will see death in terms of pathophysiology ... The obstetricians will consider that the infant died from maternal antepartum haemorrhage with its predictable complications. The pathologist tends to be impressed more by the final event than the initial one, and will attribute death to the intraventricular haemorrhage ... The epidemiologist may observe that the pregnancy could have had a different result had not the girl had such an unpromising social background. And the girl's mother, with some truth and equal conviction, will see the boyfriend as the cause of the whole unhappy episode.
(Source unknown)

Birth registration and notification and death registration allow epidemiologists to look at which groups of mothers and babies die. For example, routinely collected statistics show that two-thirds of perinatal deaths occur in the 7% of babies who weigh less than 2500 g at birth and half of all perinatal deaths in the 1% of babies who weigh less than 1500 g at birth.[4] These figures give us groups that are at risk of death and show where services could be concentrated to try to improve outcomes. But why do some very small babies survive and others die? Is it only the issue of weight? Why are some babies born too soon? What part does the mother's lifestyle play? Do maternity services both in the community and in hospital contribute to some deaths?

The medical press has recently made much of the lessons on the investigation of adverse clinical incidents that could be learnt from the aviation industry.[7] Surveys in operating theatres have confirmed that pilots and doctors have common interpersonal problem areas and similarities in professional culture.[8] These studies conclude:

Accepting the inevitability of error and the importance of reliable data on error and its management will allow systematic efforts to reduce the frequency and severity of adverse events.

Errors are due to systems rather than individuals; a good system for managing a clinical condition will minimise any risks from the mistakes of an individual – for example, checking dosages with another clinician. Many aviation schemes allow anonymous reporting of incidents so that analysis looks at systems rather than individuals. Current literature emphasizes the need for formal protocols to ensure systematic, comprehensive and efficient investigations of clinical incidents to avoid routine assignment of blame.[9] This interest in the application of industrial risk management to public services may appear to be a new development. However, clinicians in maternity services in the UK have used anonymized case reports from confidential enquiries to study maternal deaths in the UK since 1952 – a form of external clinical audit.[10]

In a confidential enquiry, details about each death are anonymized, removing the names of the unit where the event took place and of the staff involved. Some data to identify the type of unit – for example, tertiary specialist centre or district general hospital – and job titles may be included to help analysis. These details are used to complete a standardized proforma. Groups of clinicians from different disciplines concerned in maternity care meet as case assessment panels to review these proformas individually. The assessors identify those deaths associated with some aspect of care that the assessors regard as falling below the expected level of professional competence and identify 'avoidable', 'adverse' or 'notable' factors that may have contributed to the death. These may include factors about resources and the behaviour of the mother as well as the competence of the staff involved. Avoidability is extremely difficult to judge and may vary with the individual and over time. The 5th Confidential Enquiry into Stillbirths and Deaths in Infancy (CESDI) annual report[11] included a study of 'second pass' panels, a process by which the same cases were assessed by two different panels, working independently to assess consistency, which showed that there was agreement with the degree of suboptimal management in three-quarters of repeated panels – but the comments were often different. More recent CESDI programmes have used national standards to judge the quality of care. Identification of less than optimal resources and practice can be fed back anonymously to all clinicians and managers in all units to make them rethink how they provide maternity care.

Development of the Confidential Enquiry into Maternal Deaths

The main concern of obstetricians was originally for maternal rather than perinatal deaths. In 1928, the maternal mortality rate was 4.4 deaths per 1000 maternities, or 3000 mothers dying each year in England and Wales. This compares with over 41 000 babies dying at or shortly after birth in the same year (PNMR 60.8 per 1000 total births).[4] Over the next 20 years, the introduction of antibiotics, a national blood transfusion service, improved general anaesthesia and local review of deaths led to falls in maternal mortality. However, there was still wide variation in the quality and standards of both enquiry and practice in different parts of the country and between units. In response, the government set up the Confidential Enquiry into Maternal Deaths (CEMD) in 1952 (when the maternal mortality rate was 5.3 maternal deaths per 1000 maternities). Reports have been issued every 3 years since then. The Chief Medical Officer report of 1952 stated that 'CEMD's prime purpose was to place the clinical enquiries and assessment of avoidable factors in the hands of practising consultant obstetricians'. The enquiry includes deaths within 1 year of delivery or abortion and covers associated (for example, deaths due to accidents) as well as direct maternal deaths (such as deaths due to eclampsia).

Development of the national Confidential Enquiry into Stillbirths and Deaths in Infancy

Until the 1990s, there were over 100 perinatal deaths for each maternal death. Both mortality rates have fallen rapidly – there was a fourfold fall in perinatal mortality between 1956 and 1990 from 32 to 8 per 1000 births. However, there are now over 130 perinatal deaths for each mother who dies. The numbers of direct maternal deaths (about 330 a year in 1952, falling to 43 a year by 1996 – see Table 1.3) were low enough to allow individual enquiry into each case, albeit on a local level until 1952. The relatively large number of deaths of babies could only be studied through epidemiological surveys at this stage.

Three national perinatal mortality surveys were undertaken in 1946, 1958 and 1972. The first of these national studies[12] was more concerned with examining maternity services in Britain at the time when the NHS was being planned than with looking at causes of death. In 1958, the British Perinatal Mortality study[13] evaluated nationally how and when British babies were born or died, how often they died and what clinico-pathological features led to their death. The study used a cohort of births between the 3rd and 9th of March 1958, plus deaths in the next 3 consecutive months. This cohort has been studied long term to look at the effects of prenatal factors in parents on the next generation.[14] The detailed first report contained statistical data on factors such as maternal age, parity, place of booking, gestation and birthweight, while the second report[15] used multivariate analysis of high-risk influences on the outcome of pregnancy, such as smoking and socio-biological factors.

A third study was done in 1970 to look at all babies born alive or dead after the 24th week of gestation.[16] This provided basic data in Britain for factors such as low birthweight and placental abnormalities

Table 1.3 Direct maternal mortality rates and perinatal mortality 1952–99

Year	Total maternities	Direct maternal deaths	Direct maternal mortality rate/100 000 maternities	Perinatal mortality rate/1000 total births	
1952–54	2052 953	1094	53.3	1954	44.5
1961–63	2520 420	692	27.5	1963	29.3
1973–75	1921 569	235	12.2	1975	19.3
1976–78	1748 849	227	13.0	1978	15.5
1979–81	1942 859	178	9.2	1981	11.8
1982–84	1883 753	138	7.3	1984	10.1
1985–87	2293 508	139	6.1	1987	8.9
1988–90	2374 800	145	6.1	1990	8.1
1991–93	2346 800	128	5.6	1993	9.0*
1994–96	2197 640	134	6.1	1996	8.3*
				1999	8.2*

*Includes stillbirths 24–27 weeks gestational age
Source: Confidential Enquiries into Maternal Deaths reports and ONS statistics.

and quantified them. These studies did not look at deaths individually but epidemiologically. A proposed fourth study in 1982 did not occur in England and Wales.[17] By this time, perinatal deaths had fallen to a level (12 per 1000 total births or over 7000 deaths a year) where it was possible to do a confidential enquiry on a proportion of deaths. A more unified routine data-collection system for the far fewer births taking place in Scotland made a Scottish study on each death feasible at this time.[18,19]

Despite falls in the UK PNMR, comparisons of the perinatal mortality rates between Western countries in the 1970s led the Committee on Child Health Services in 1976[20] to refer to the infant mortality rate in the UK as a 'holocaust'.

We have failed to keep pace with many other countries in our effort to make birth and the first months of life a less dangerous time.

Of every thousand births occurring in England and Wales, 11 are still born; of every thousand live born, 11 die in the first four weeks and 16 fail to survive their first year.

In contemporary terms infant mortality is a holocaust, equal to all deaths in the succeeding 24 years of life.[19]

In 1973, the PNMR for England and Wales was 21.5 per 1000 births compared to 18 in Japan and 14 in Sweden. Within the UK, there were also wide variations in PNMRs – 21 per 1000 total births in West Midlands region to 14 in East Anglia – that needed investigation. Several English regions (Northern, South East Thames, Wessex, and Mersey) started confidential enquiries in the late 1970s. Some involved interviews with the bereaved parents and the primary care professionals involved to discover the parents' view of what went wrong in the pregnancy and their views on how staff helped them to cope with their loss.[21–24] These studies have been instrumental in improving the quality of bereavement support for parents.

Stillbirth and neonatal mortality rates fell particularly quickly in the late 1970s and early 1980s. In England and Wales, the PNMR fell by 48% from 19.3 in 1975 to 10.1 per thousand by 1985. There are now equal proportions of stillbirths to early neonatal deaths but this was not always the case. In the 1930s the stillbirth rate was more than double the first week death rate. Stillbirth and early neonatal death rates began to converge in the mid 1950s, reaching the same levels by the mid 1970s. This is similar to trends in other Western countries, which are all beginning to converge at rates of less than 10 per 1000. However, there was a marked flattening of the rate of fall of late neonatal and post-neonatal mortality rates between 1976 and the late 1980s. The final political incentive for a confidential enquiry into stillbirths and deaths in infancy came in 1986 when the infant mortality rate rose to 9.6 from 9.4 per thousand the previous year. (This is likely to have been due to an increase in sudden unexplained deaths in infancy.) A House of Commons Social Services Committee enquiry called for a targeted programme – the government response was to require all English regions, Northern Ireland and Wales to set up full stillbirth and infant death surveys from 1 January 1993 as part of the national programme. The failure to establish an integrated national system from the start meant that CESDI inherited disparate regional systems that needed to be systematized over its first few years. However, the strong regional basis helps to ensure good case ascertainment and good feedback of CESDI findings to clinicians locally.

Slightly contrary to its name, CESDI covers all deaths from the 20th week of pregnancy to the end of the first year of life, including some late fetal losses as well as all stillbirths. Scotland has a separate survey of stillbirths and neonatal deaths.[25] The death is notified to a local co-ordinator who notifies the regional office using a rapid report form (RRF). RRFs for all included deaths are used to find cases for enquiry and supply a limited set of epidemiological data. Statutory returns on all births and deaths supply a considerable amount of relevant data to put these deaths into overall context.[26,27] However, without good denominator data from detailed information on all births or a proper case-control study, it is impossible to put perinatal deaths in an enquiry into perspective and calculate a relative risk for factors leading to perinatal death.[28] This is a major problem of current confidential enquiries. Adverse factors occur in the care of mothers and babies who survive as well as those who die. Lack of denominator data to put the risks in perspective makes it impossible to assess the sensitivity and specificity of screening for adverse risk factors. Most screening tests in pregnancy produce a high proportion of false positives, leading to unnecessary clinical intervention, and there is a danger that confidential enquiries may contribute to this if no effort is made to look at the overall background. For example, the focus group looking at breech presentation at the onset of labour[29] studied 56 cases of normally formed babies weighing over 1.5 kg who died during labour or delivery, and who presented by the breech. Thirty-two of these babies were undiagnosed breeches. Without denominator data for all undiagnosed breech presentations, it is impossible to calculate the risk of death for a baby who has not been diagnosed as a breech. Further in-depth discussion about babies who presented as breech presentations may be found in Chapter 6.

Studies of sudden infant deaths with controls were undertaken in three regions as a pilot study for the national CESDI to look at the use of case controls in assessing adverse factors.[30] This topic is covered in full in Chapter 7.

Controls were used in the 1998–2000 CESDI study of deaths (Project 27/28) in babies born at 27 or 28 weeks' gestation.[31] These findings are highlighted in Chapter 5.

RECENT INTERNATIONAL COMPARISONS

The initial response to low ratings for the UK in international 'league tables' was the setting up of confidential enquiries into perinatal deaths. An international confidential enquiry gives some clues as to how the UK ranks since the introduction of national CESDI and how difficult it is to judge suboptimal care. The Euronatal study identified perinatal deaths between 1993 and 1998 in regions of ten European countries.[32,33] An international audit panel using explicit audit criteria reviewed cases of fetal deaths (28 weeks or more), intrapartum deaths (28 or more weeks) and neonatal deaths (34 or more weeks), excluding deaths with major congenital malformations. Cases were anonymized for region.

The audit covered 1619 cases of perinatal deaths, representing 90% of eligible cases in the regions. Consensus was reached in 95% of cases. In 4%, suboptimal factors, which possibly or probably had contributed to the fatal outcome, were identified. The percentage of cases with such suboptimal factors was significantly lower in the Finnish and Swedish regions compared with the remaining regions of Spain, the Netherlands, Scotland, Belgium, Denmark, Norway, Greece and England. Failure to detect severe intrauterine growth retardation (IUGR) (10%) and smoking in combination with severe IUGR and/or placental abruption (12%) were the most frequent suboptimal factors. There was positive association between the proportion of suboptimal factors and the overall PMR in the regions. This was a large study using national and international panels to judge whether care was suboptimal. Only 4% of cases were judged to be unauditable from the data given, but such a complex methodology will inevitably have some variability between and within different panels.

CONFIDENTIAL ENQUIRIES INTO STILLBIRTHS AND DEATHS IN INFANCY PROGRAMMES

CESDI provides an overview of the numbers and causes of stillbirth and infant deaths, with detailed enquiries into specific sub-sets. CESDI has used case-control studies where risk factors need to be assessed and focus-group work to provide detail and overview of rare events.

The confidential enquiry process requires assessments of anonymized case notes by local multidisciplinary regional panels of obstetricians, paediatricians, midwives, GPs, neonatal nurses, pathologists, public-health doctors and others. The panels are selected to be geographically separate from the cases and are not involved in the care of these babies. Lay groups have put the case that the panels should also include lay members, but this has not yet happened. The numbers of deaths are still too great for every death to be reviewed by the enquiry process, although every death is recorded via the RRF.

Different subgroups were targeted for a more detailed investigation by peer review panels in each part of the programme. Table 1.4 shows the different subgroups that have been studied. The initial subgroup for confidential enquiry kept the CESDI focus on maternity services by auditing intrapartum-related deaths of normally formed babies of birth weight greater than 2500 g. This focussed on babies who would be expected to have developed beyond the stage when the problems of prematurity might influence their survival. The definitions were extended in 1995 to include babies who met the

Table 1.4   The CESDI work programme 1993–99

	Year of study	Findings reported
Enquiry topic		
Methods and results	1993	1st annual report
Sudden unexpected deaths in infancy	1993–4	3rd annual report
Intrapartum related deaths >2.5 kg	1993	2nd annual report
Intrapartum related deaths >1.5 kg	1994–5	4th annual report
'Explained' sudden unexpected deaths in infancy	1993–6	5th annual report
'1 in 10' sample of all deaths >1 kg	1996–7	6th annual report
All deaths 4 kg and over	1997	6th annual report
Case control studies		
Sudden unexpected deaths in infancy	1993–6	3rd and 5th annual report
Antepartum term stillbirths	1995	5th annual report
Project 27/28	1998–2000	8th annual report
Focus groups and central reviews		
Shoulder dystocia	1994–5	5th annual report
Ruptured uterus	1994–5	5th annual report
Planned home delivery	1994–5	5th annual report
Anaesthetic complications and delays	1994–5	7th annual report
Breech presentation at onset of labour	1994–5	7th annual report
Stillbirths	1996–7	8th annual report
Audits and collaborative work		
Postmortem reporting	1993, 1994–5	2nd and 8th annual report
CTG education	1999	7th annual report
European comparisons of perinatal care	1995–8	7th annual report
Use of electronic fetal monitoring	1999	8th annual report

Copies of CESDI reports from the 5th report onwards are available from the website:
http://www.cesdi.org.uk/CESDIpublications.htm
or http://www.cemach.org.uk/publicationstemp.html

following criteria. An intrapartum death was defined as the death after the onset of labour and before 28 days of life of a normally formed baby weighing 1.5 kg or more related to intrapartum events. This group of 873 babies (1 in every 1561 births) represented only 4.3% of CESDI deaths, but was felt to be the group that was most amenable to improvement through feedback of the organizational problems in maternity care identified in the national CESDI reports.

Over 78% of these intrapartum-related deaths were criticized for suboptimal care because alternative management 'might' (25%) or 'would reasonably be expected to' (52%) have made a difference to the outcome. About 95% of critical comments described failures to act appropriately, to recognize problems or to communicate effectively. The dominant time for suboptimal care was during labour (70% of comments), followed by antepartum (19%) and post partum (11%), with 22% of the 375 neonatal deaths having suboptimal resuscitation.[34]

Other CESDI reports include confidential enquiries on a 1 in 10 sample of all deaths over 1 kg (excluding post neonatal deaths and major abnormalities), and all deaths of babies of 4 kg or over. Reports from focus groups cover shoulder dystocia, ruptured uterus, planned home delivery, anaesthetic complications and delays, and breech presentation at the onset of labour.[10, 28, 35] The last CESDI study was on diabetic pregnancies.

USING THE RESULTS OF CONFIDENTIAL ENQUIRIES INTO MATERNAL DEATHS, STILLBIRTHS AND DEATHS IN INFANCY

Untoward outcomes in maternity care have huge costs, emotionally to families and economically to the NHS. The NHS Litigation Authority is a special health authority that indemnifies and manages claims on NHS bodies for clinical negligence and non-clinical risks. One in five claims relates to obstetrics, which costs 80% of all claims, with awards of up to £3.5 million. It is, therefore, vital that risks are identified through CEMD and CESDI and trusts change practice to tackle them. Clinicians take the task of learning from their mistakes very seriously. There is no statutory requirement to take part in CEMD or CESDI, but ascertainment of cases reported by comparison with registered deaths suggests that very few cases indeed are not included in the confidential enquiries.

Passively providing information about the results of research and feedback on individual practice is unlikely to produce change unless it is linked to audit and educational processes.[36] It is, therefore, important that feedback from confidential enquiries is active. In the late 1980s, there was concern that CEMD was not producing change as it relied on passive feedback of pooled anonymous data, and recently there have been efforts to ensure that recommendations in the reports are acted on, and protocols for dealing with potentially fatal complications are available.[37] Publishing reports is not enough – CESDI has also undertaken audits on post mortem reporting, cardiotocograph education and resuscitation of premature babies to see if messages from its reports are noted and changes implemented.

It has also produced notes for both parents and professionals on post mortem examination to encourage both the offer and the uptake. This is essential if the causes of perinatal deaths are to be determined accurately so that action can be taken to prevent future deaths. Regional CESDI coordinators have worked hard in their own localities to feed back CEMD and CESDI findings as an aid to continuing professional development. A national incentive to implement the recommendations from CESDI and CEMD reports came in 2001.

The Clinical Negligence Scheme for Trusts (CNST) is a voluntary risk pooling scheme set up under Section 21 of the National Health Service and Community Care Act 1990[37] to help NHS trusts manage their clinical negligence liabilities. It is self-funding through annual contributions from member trusts, assessed according to the type of services the trust provides and their past claims history. Achievement of the CNST risk management standards by trusts means that they are putting into place systems for ensuring that the quality of health care is maintained and improved, and reducing the scope for clinical negligence claims – and their contribution is discounted according to their level of compliance with the eight core maternity standards. In 2001, CNST required 'Evidence of Trust Board or Governance Group review of recommendations from the National Confidential Enquiries' as part of their 'Standard 1 – lessons from experience'.[38]

FUTURE PROGRAMMES

CEMD and CESDI were initially run as separate enquiries by the Department of Health. Changes in the NHS meant that in 1999 the National Institute for Clinical Excellence (NICE) received responsibility for the four national confidential enquiries; CEMD (established in 1952), CESDI (established in 1993), the National Confidential Enquiry into Perioperative Deaths (NCEPOD) (established in 1988) and the Confidential Inquiry into Suicide and Homicide by People with Mental Illness (CISH) (established in 1991). NICE took this opportunity for a review of all the confidential enquiries and decided to merge CEMD and CESDI into a larger enquiry with a wider remit – looking at deaths of pregnant women, late fetal losses, stillbirths and children up to the age of 16 years. The new Confidential Enquiry into Maternal and Child Health (CEMACH) was launched in April 2003. CEMACH will retain its regional base.

CEMACH is funded through NICE and is managed by a Consortium of Royal Colleges, which includes the Royal College of

Obstetricians and Gynaecologists, the Royal College of Midwives, the Royal College of Paediatrics and Child Health, the Royal College of Pathologists, the Royal College of Anaesthetists and the Faculty of Public Health. In 2004, a scoping study for a confidential enquiry into childhood deaths will start, aiming to establish:

- the practical issues associated with data collection and panel formation for enquiries into childhood deaths
- potential areas for study through the confidential enquiry method based on initial findings from trial panel enquiries
- worthwhile topics and recommendations for study at a national level.

KEY MESSAGES

- Routinely collected data from statutory birth registration and notification supply birth rates and allow epidemiological study of births. It cannot provide detailed analysis of the causes of deaths relating deaths to how clinicians practice, provision of maternity services or women's social circumstances.

- Concern about deaths of pregnant women led to the CEMD in 1952 – the first of its kind in the world. Political and professional concern about the deaths of babies, especially in comparison with other countries, led to the development of local confidential enquiries into stillbirths and deaths in infancy in the late 1970s and 1980s and to national CESDI in 1993.

- Confidential enquiries aim to improve clinical practice through the investigation of deaths in specific circumstances, with panels assessing anonymized, standardized case histories against national standards. Confidential enquiries look at how systems (both clinical and social) fail mothers and babies, and do not look at the role of individuals.

- Lessons learnt from confidential enquiries must be communicated through the professions and through risk management and clinical governance in maternity services.

ACKNOWLEDGEMENTS

ONS statistics on mortality rates from Macfarlane A, Mugford M 2000 Birth counts: statistics of pregnancy and childbirth. The Stationery Office, London

References

1. Lewis G, Drife J (eds) 2001 Why mothers die 1997–1999, the fifth report of the confidential enquiries into maternal deaths in the United Kingdom. Royal College of Obstetricians and Gynaecologists Press, London
2. Peller S 1948 Mortality past and future. Population Studies 1: 405–456
3. Nissel M 1987 People count; a history of the general register office. HMSO, London
4. Macfarlane A, Mugford M 2000 Birth counts: statistics of pregnancy and childbirth. The Stationery Office, London
5. Keirse MJNC 1984 Perinatal mortality rates do not contain what they purport to contain. Lancet i: 1166–1169
6. Fenton AC, Field DJ, Mason E, Clarke M 1990 Attitudes to viability of preterm infants and their effect on figures for perinatal mortality. British Medical Journal 300: 434–436
7. Helmreich R 2000 On error management: lessons from aviation. British Medical Journal 320: 781–785
8. Sexton JB, Thomas EJ, Helmreich RL 2000 Error, stress, and teamwork in medicine and aviation: cross sectional surveys. British Medical Journal 320: 745–749
9. Vincent C, Taylor-Adams S, Chapman J et al. 2000 How to investigate and analyse clinical incidents: clinical risk unit and association of litigation and risk management protocol. British Medical Journal 320: 777–781
10. Shaw CD 1980 Aspects of audit. British Medical Journal 1: 1256
11. Maternal and Child Health Research Consortium 1998 CESDI, 5th annual report. Department of Health, London
12. Joint Committee of the Royal College of Obstetrics and Gynaecology and the British Paediatric Association 1949 Neonatal mortality and morbidity. Reports on Public Health and Medical Subjects No. 94. HMSO, London
13. Butler NR, Bonham DG 1963 Perinatal mortality. The first report of the 1958 British perinatal mortality survey. E&S Livingstone, Edinburgh
14. Emanuel I, Filakati H, Alberman E, Evans SJW 1992 Intergenerational studies of human birthweight from the 1958 birth cohort.1. Evidence for a multigenerational effect. British Journal of Obstetrics and Gynaecology 99: 67–74
15. Butler NR, Alberman ED (eds) 1969 Perinatal problems: the second report of the 1958 British perinatal mortality survey. E&S Livingstone, Edinburgh
16. Chamberlain R, Chamberlain G, Howlett B, Claireaux A 1975 The first week of life. British births 1970, vol 1. Butterworth Heinemann Medical, London
17. Chalmers I 1979 Desirability and feasibility of a 4th national perinatal survey: report submitted to the Children's and Reproductive Research Liaison Group's Research Division of the DHSS. National Perinatal Epidemiology Unit, Oxford
18. McIlwaine GM, Howat RCL, Dunn F, MacNaughton MC 1979 The Scottish perinatal mortality survey. British Medical Journal 2: 1103–1106

19. Chalmers I, McIlwaine G (eds) 1980 Perinatal audit and surveillance. Proceedings of the 8th study group. Royal College of Obstetricians and Gynaecologists, London

20. Committee on Child Health Services 1976 Fit for the future. Cmnd 6684 (Court report). HMSO, London

21. Paediatric Research Unit, Royal Devon and Exeter Hospital 1973 A suggested model for inquiries into perinatal and early childhood deaths in a health care district. Children's Research Fund Report

22. Mersey Region Working Party on Perinatal Mortality 1982 Confidential inquiry into perinatal deaths in the Mersey region. Lancet i: 491–494

23. Mutch LMM, Brown NJ, Spiedel BD, Dunn PM 1981 Perinatal mortality and neonatal survival in Avon: 1976–79. British Medical Journal 282: 119–122

24. Wood B, Catford JC, Cogswell JJ 1984 Confidential paediatric enquiry into neonatal deaths in Wessex, 1981 and 1982. British Medical Journal 288: 1206–1208

25. Information and Statistics Division 1993 The National Health Service in Scotland. Scottish Stillbirth and Neonatal Death Report 1993. Common Services Agency, ISD Publications, Edinburgh

26. Black N, Macfarlane A 1982 Methodological kit: monitoring mortality statistics in a health district. Community Medicine 4: 25–33

27. Clarke M 1982 Perinatal audit: a tried and tested epidemiological method. Community Medicine 4: 104–107

28. Coggon D, Rose R, Barker DJP 1993 Epidemiology for the uninitiated. British Medical Journal, London

29. Maternal and Child Health Research Consortium 2000 CESDI 7th annual report. Department of Health, London

30. Fleming P, Blair P, Bacon C, Berry J 2000 Sudden unexpected deaths in infancy; the CESDI SUDI studies 1993–96. The Stationery Office, London

31. Confidential Enquiries into Stillbirths and Deaths in Infancy 2003 Project 27–28. The Stationery Office, Norwich

32. Richardus JH, Wilco C, Graafmans et al. 2002 Differences in perinatal mortality and suboptimal care between ten European regions: results of an international audit. British Journal of Obstetrics and Gynaecology 110: 97–105

33. Maternal and Child Health Research Consortium 2001 CESDI 8th annual report. Department of Health, London

34. Maternal and Child Health Research Consortium 1997 CESDI 4th annual report. Department of Health, London

35. Maternal and Child Health Research Consortium 1999 CESDI 6th annual report. Department of Health, London

36. Mugford M, Banfield P, O'Hanlon M 1991 The effects of feedback of information on clinical practice: a review. British Medical Journal 303: 398–402

37. Patel N (ed.) 1992 Maternal mortality – the way forward. Royal College of Obstetricians and Gynaecologists, London

38. *http://www.nhsla.com/Welcome_to_NHSLA.htm*

Chapter **2**

History of the confidential enquiries into maternal deaths

Gwyneth Lewis

Whose faces are behind the numbers? What were their stories? What were their dreams? They left behind children and families. They also left behind clues as to why their lives end so early.[1]

GLOBAL PICTURE

The UK and other developed countries, unlike many parts of the world, have low maternal mortality rates. Globally, each year, approximately eight million women suffer pregnancy-related complications and over half a million will die.[2] In developing countries 1 in 11 women may die of pregnancy-related complications, compared to 1 in 5000 in developed countries. Each death or long-term complication represents an individual tragedy for the woman, her partner, her children and family. More tragically, most are avoidable. The main causes are haemorrhage, sepsis, eclampsia and unsafe abortion, and more than 80% of maternal deaths could be prevented or avoided through actions that are proven to be effective and affordable, even in the poorer countries of the world.

While the overall global maternal mortality rate is 27 deaths per 100 000 live births, in many developing countries it is nearly 20 times higher, at between 500 and 600 deaths per 100 000 live births. Unfortunately, in a few countries, mainly in Africa, it is even higher, reaching figures greater than 1000/100 000 births.[2] The rates of many of the developing countries with average maternal mortality rates still far exceed those in the UK over 100 years ago. Women in these countries die usually because they are not provided with the health care that they need, either through a lack of basic facilities or through an inability to access the local healthcare services. Only 53% of women in developing countries receive assistance from a skilled attendant at birth. Some women are denied access to care because of cultural practices of seclusion or because responsibility for decision making falls to other family members. In some cases, the failure of support for pregnant women by families, partners or their government also reflects the societal value placed on women's lives. Thus, in developing countries, the overwhelming risk factor for maternal mortality is the lack of access, for whatever reason, to even basic education or clinical or public health care. Addressing these inequalities and reducing the maternal mortality in these countries is a leading priority for the World Health Organization (WHO).

Looking beyond the numbers

The numbers of global maternal mortality are stark enough but they tell only part of the story. In particular, they tell us nothing about the *faces behind the numbers*, the individual stories of suffering and distress and the real underlying reasons why mothers die. Most of all, they tell us nothing about why women continue to die in a world where the knowledge and resources to prevent such deaths are available or attainable. While it is important to keep monitoring overall levels of maternal mortality at global, regional and national levels, for both identification and advocacy purposes, simple statistics about the level of maternal mortality do not help identify what can be done to prevent or avoid such unnecessary deaths.

In order to help address this, the WHO's Making Pregnancy Safer strategy is shortly to publish *Beyond the Numbers*,[3] a book which describes a number of strategies and approaches to help understand why mothers die. A key component of the book is the use of Confidential Enquiries into Maternal Deaths (CEMD).

Confidential enquiries are essentially observational studies, using qualitative and quantitative analysis, which take account of the medical, and sometimes non-medical, factors that led to a woman's death. They provide data on individual cases, which when aggregated together can show trends or common factors for which remediable action may be possible. They 'tell the story' of how individual women died.

UK CONFIDENTIAL ENQUIRY INTO MATERNAL DEATHS: THE FIRST 50 YEARS

The longest running example of a CEMD is that of the UK. During the 1920s, at a time when other health indicators such as infant mortality were improving, healthcare professionals and women's advocacy groups became concerned about the apparent lack of similar improvement in levels of maternal mortality. Consequently, in 1928, local health professionals started a system of case review audits. Although not national in scope, these maternal death audits included a detailed review of adverse events. Over time, as commitment improved, these small-scale reviews or local facility audits evolved, by 1935, to wider area health authority-based systems of confidential enquiries, the recommendations of which played a major part in reducing the maternal mortality rate over the next two decades.

In commenting on the impact of the findings of these earlier enquiries, Sir George Godber, a past Chief Medical Officer for England, stated:

All this procedure had been intended to do was to secure improvements by the local review of cases, but it was soon apparent that avoidable factors were too often present in antenatal and intranatal care for the opportunity for central remediable action to be ignored.[4]

This led to the decision to undertake a national confidential enquiry for England and Wales in 1952, which was extended to cover the UK (UK CEMD) in 1985, and this is the system that is still running, and improving maternal health care, 50 years later on.

Perhaps one of the most important features of the UK CEMD reports is that they have always included anonymized 'vignettes', short case summaries that 'tell the story'. The enquiry team never forgets that each woman's death is an individual personal and family tragedy. Neither do they forget she had a unique story to tell, and tracing her path through the healthcare system and describing the remediable action that might have been taken to prevent the woman's death has a powerful effect on those who read the stories, many of whom report immediate changes in their practice as a result.

Participating in a confidential enquiry, either by providing data and writing up the history of a woman whose face and family can still be remembered, or even by assessing the case anonymously, can be regarded as a legitimate healthcare intervention. Also, as a result, personal or local changes in practice based on this experience may occur long before the report and its recommendations are published. In the UK, as long ago as 1954, it was recognized that participating in a confidential enquiry had a 'powerful secondary effect' in that 'each participant in these enquiries, however experienced he or she may be, and whether his or her work is undertaken in a teaching hospital, a local hospital, in the community or the patient's home must have benefited from their educative effect'.[5] Personal experience is, therefore, as much, or even more of a valuable tool for harnessing change as anonymous statistical reporting.

UK CONFIDENTIAL ENQUIRY INTO MATERNAL DEATHS 1997–99

The main causes of deaths in the latest report of the UK CEMD[6] are shown in Figure 2.1 and the rates shown in Table 2.1. The leading cause of maternal death directly attributable to pregnancy was pulmonary embolism, a cause that does not even appear in the list for developing countries. A record linkage study with the Office for National Statistics (ONS) showed that, overall, suicide was the leading cause of maternal death, although these were not often

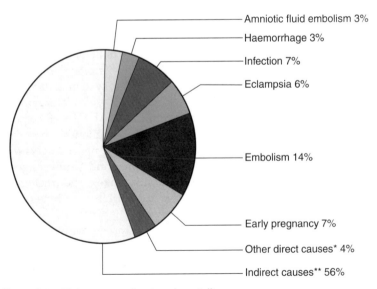

Figure 2.1   Major causes of maternal mortality

reported to the enquiry, as the death usually took place after contact with the maternity services had ceased.

During the triennium 378 deaths were reported to or identified by the enquiry, a number remarkably similar to the 376 cases reported in 1994–96. The enquiry includes deaths directly related to pregnancy (*direct*), those due to pre-exisiting disease aggravated by pregnancy (*indirect*), those in which the cause was unrelated to pregnancy (*coincidental, formally fortuitous*), and those occurring after the internationally defined limit of 6 weeks after delivery, but before 1 year from delivery (*late* deaths).[5]

Of the 378 deaths, 106 were classified as *direct* and 136 as *indirect* deaths, representing 28% and 36% of reported cases respectively. Twenty-nine (8%) were classified as *coincidental* (*fortuitous*) and 107

Table 2.1   Death rates by major cause of death per million maternities: UK 1985–99

Cause	Rate				
	1985–87	1988–90	1991–93	1994–96	1997–99
Thromboembolism	14.1	14.0	15.1	21.8	16.5
Pregnancy induced hypertension	11.9	11.4	8.6	9.1	7.1
Haemorrhage	4.4	9.3	6.5	5.5	3.3
Amniotic fluid embolism	4.0	4.7	4.3	7.7	3.8
Early pregnancy	7.9*	7.6*	5.2*	6.8	8.0
Sepsis	4.4	5.5	6.4	6.4*	6.6*
Total uterine trauma/other	11.9	7.2	6.0	3.2	3.3
Direct					
– Uterine trauma	2.6	1.3	1.7	2.3	1.0
– Other *direct*	9.3	5.9	4.3	0.9	2.3
Anaesthetic	2.6	1.7	3.5	0.5	1.4
Cardiac *indirect*	10.1	7.6	15.9	17.7	16.5
Psychiatric *indirect***	–	–	–	4.1	7.1
Other *indirect*	37.0	31.0	27.0	39.1	35.3
Indirect maligancies					5.1
Total *direct* and *indirect*	98.2	100.1	98.1	121.9	11.4
Coincidental (fortuitous)	11.3	16.5	19.9	16.4	10.8
Late	N/A	20.3	19.9	32.8	50.3

*Including sepsis in early pregnancy; **until 1993–96 counted as coincidental

(28%) as *late*. In this triennium the total number of *direct* and *indirect* maternal deaths reported to the enquiry, 242, is lower than the 268 reported in the previous triennium. However, for the first time the number of *indirect* deaths exceeded the number of *direct* deaths.

Maternal deaths are the tip of the iceberg of maternal morbidity and reducing the risk factors for maternal deaths should also reduce the numbers of women who experience significant medical or psycho-logical problems during or after birth, sometimes with long-lasting or permanent sequelae. A number of studies have been published on the incidence of severe maternal morbidity, or 'near-misses', but comparison between them is difficult because of the inclusion criteria used. The death to near-miss ratio in these studies ranges from 1:5[7] to 1:118.[8]

Vulnerability and risk factors for maternal deaths

The UK CEMD has been increasingly widening its scope with the aim of identifying further possible risk factors for maternal deaths in order to improve services for pregnant and recently delivered women. The latest report, because of the development of sophisticated coding programmes with ONS, was, for the first time, able to evaluate more fully any social and lifestyle factors that may have contributed to the woman's death. These findings cause great concern, showing the maternal mortality rates among the socially excluded, including women from lower socio-economic classes, very young girls and specific ethnic groups, to be very much higher than those among the population as a whole. A summary of the findings shows that:

- women from the most disadvantaged groups of society are about 20 times more likely to die than women in the highest two social classes
- non-white women are, on average, twice as likely to die as white women; many of these women spoke little English
- in many cases, professionals used family members to interpret; there were several difficult cases where children were used inappropriately to interpret intimate personal or social details of the mother and vital information was withheld
- a disproportionate number of women from the traditional travelling community were likely to die
- 12% of all the women whose deaths are included in the report declared that they were subject to violence in the home
- 30% of the women who died had booked for maternity care after 24 weeks of gestation or had missed over four routine antenatal visits.

Other factors are also associated with an increased risk of death, for example, very young mothers, increasing maternal age over 35 and parity. Many women whose deaths were considered by the enquiry were also obese and/or smoked.

Pre-existing maternal ill health

In the UK, *indirect* deaths from complications arising from pre-existing medical or psychological disease now outnumber those from obstetric causes. This underlines the significant contribution that coexisting maternal physical or psychological co-morbidity can have on pregnancy outcome for both mother and child. Women with significant disease benefit from personalized multidisciplinary antenatal care, for example through combined diabetic, epileptic or cardiac clinics, or through a referral to an obstetric physician. The provision of flexible multidisciplinary services for women at risk from mental illness or substance misuse is also of significant importance.

Guidelines work

The results of CEMD reports show, sometimes in dramatic fashion, that the routine use of national guidelines can work. In this triennium, following the routine introduction and use of guidelines developed, in part, as a result of findings and recommendations from previous CEMD reports, there have been significant decreases in deaths from pulmonary embolism and sepsis following Caesarean section. In the very few cases where deaths occurred from these causes, guidelines do not appear to have been followed.

Substandard care

Substandard care was difficult to evaluate in some of the cases in this report due to the lack of key data from some records and case notes. Whilst it is clear that many of the cases received less than optimum care it has not always been possible to quantify these with certainty. Nevertheless, despite these limitations, the assessors classified 60.4% of *direct* deaths as having involved some form of substandard care. Fifty per cent of *direct* deaths had involved major substandard care, in which different treatment may have affected the outcome. Seventeen per cent of *indirect* deaths and 9% of deaths from cardiac disease were associated with substandard care. By contrast only about 10% of both *coincidental* and *late* deaths had substandard care, with 7% in each category being classified as major. The major concerns about the care of these cases were related to failings in social service support for vulnerable young girls and to the lack of multidisciplinary or co-ordinated care.

The main causes of substandard care can be summarized as:

- lack of communication and team work
- failure to appreciate the severity of the illness and suboptimal treatment
- wrong diagnoses
- failure of junior staff or general practitioners (GPs) to diagnose or refer the case to a senior colleague or hospital
- failure of consultants to attend, and inappropriate delegation of responsibility
- in some units, the continuing lack of a clear policy for the prevention or treatment of conditions such as pulmonary embolism, eclampsia or massive haemorrhage
- failure of the lead professional to identify diseases or conditions that do not commonly occur in their own specialty, or to seek early advice.

OVERALL THEMES IN RELATION TO MIDWIFERY PRACTICE

Midwives provide the majority of care and are frequently the lead healthcare practitioner for pregnant and recently delivered women. With increasing emphasis on midwifery-led care, this latter role will continue to expand. Even when midwives are not the lead practitioner they continue to see most women during their pregnancy, delivery and the postnatal period. Midwives are the professional lead for approximately 70% of births and are involved in the remaining 30%, which are usually higher-risk deliveries.[9] Although many women in this report had higher-risk pregnancies, complications or underlying medical conditions that required specialist obstetric or multidisciplinary care, midwives were also involved in their care. In most cases midwives provided the important continuity, supportive link and point of contact between the woman and a number of different healthcare professionals. In some cases midwives were also the healthcare professional who picked up the early signs of possible complications and referred the woman for appropriate care.

All but 21 of the 378 women whose deaths are included in the report had had contact with the midwifery services. The 21 who had no contact died before booking or after a miscarriage or termination of pregnancy. A total of eight women had midwifery-led care, and a further 42 had joint midwifery/GP-led care. One hundred and ninety received 'traditional' shared care, and 56, who had high-risk pregnancies, were cared for solely in the hospital setting.

From the detailed assessment four key themes emerged in relation to midwifery practice:

1. Appropriate provision and targeting of care
2. Professional accountability and responsibility, including advocacy
3. Risk assessment
4. Communication.

These themes are presented here as separate areas for discussion, but they are interwoven and share many similarities and common threads.

In addition, the latest report contains valuable new information for midwives and other health professionals, for example, in relation to mental illness and thromboprophylaxis. Specific clinical recommendations relevant to midwifery practice taken from the relevant chapters in the main report or in the midwifery or executive summary can also be found at *www.cemd.org.uk.*

Appropriate provision and targeting of care

Each woman is an individual with different social, physical and emotional needs as well as having specific clinical factors that may affect her pregnancy. Her pregnancy should not be viewed in isolation from other important factors that may influence her health or that of her developing baby.

Midwives have a unique role in providing the majority of antenatal care and are well placed to address health inequalities and health-promotion issues. *Making a Difference*[10] suggests that midwives should target vulnerable groups who would not traditionally use the health-promotion services. In this triennium, however, midwives appear to have missed some opportunities to do so and there were many instances where women appeared to be just slotted into a rigid antenatal-care programme that was inflexible and inappropriate for their specific needs.

Social exclusion

The midwife has a vital role to play, not only in contributing to the health and well-being of all mothers and their babies, but also in targeting their care to those mothers most in need. Socio-economic deprivation was a prominent factor in a large number of cases considered by this report, and was associated with a tendency to delay access to, or attend regularly for midwifery care.

Five girls aged 16 years or less, and a total of 13 women aged 18 years or less died in this triennium. All but one were severely socially excluded. Four of the five girls aged less than 16 years had been in the care of social services, and three of these girls were homeless and living 'rough' at the time of their death. All but one of the deaths in women aged between 16 and 18 years were also characterized by social exclusion. Seven had suffered repeated episodes of domestic violence from within their own family and several of these also had suffered sexual abuse.

All women should have equal access to information and advice regardless of their social circumstances or how articulate they are. Whilst mothers who live in more deprived circumstances constitute a specific at-risk group, it is important to adopt an individual approach to needs assessment, tailoring the care given to the specific circumstances of each mother. Examples of appropriate targeting of care in specific circumstances are discussed below. Hart et al.[11] concluded that midwives who work with disadvantaged clients need to be able to understand a woman's social and cultural background, act as an advocate with medical staff and colleagues, and overcome their own prejudices and practise in a reflective manner.

The booking visit presents an opportunity to undertake a complete, holistic, needs assessment of the woman. This should include identification of factors relating to social exclusion, including problems such as learning difficulties.

Poor attenders at antenatal clinic and/or women who booked late

Twenty per cent of the total number of women who died from *direct* and *indirect* causes in this enquiry either booked after 20 weeks of pregnancy or missed more than four or more antenatal visits. Whilst it is not possible to follow-up women who are unknown to the service, it was clear in many instances that non-attendance in women who had booked generated a routine appointment by post. It is not known if this was purely an administrative response or whether professionals were involved. Further, it is not clear if this decision was made based on information in the maternity records. Midwives should be aware of their professional responsibility in the protection of the interests of the mother and her baby, ensuring that they are central to the delivery of care.

Targeting care is about developing services that are effective for all women but particularly for those women who would not normally actively seek help and advice. As part of the changes in the delivery of midwifery care it is crucial that new patterns of antenatal care are developed particularly for those women who are at the greatest risk. In some instances this may require individual antenatal care at home.

Nearly half of the women who booked after 20 weeks of pregnancy, or who were poor attenders at antenatal clinics, came from ethnic-minority groups. Half of these women did not speak English. In some cases midwives did go into the community to follow these women up, but in others either no active follow-up was undertaken or letters were sent in English advising the woman to attend her next appointment. There were several instances of such letters not being understood by any family member.

Ethnicity

Issues to do with late booking and poor attendance in these groups of women have been discussed in the preceding section. There were also many mothers in this triennium who spoke little or no English. In all of these groups language difficulties and lack of knowledge of specific cultural practices may have led to a lack of understanding, which may have contributed to the midwife not being aware of critical signs and symptoms. In some cases midwives asked relatives, who themselves did not speak much English, to contact the GP because the midwife was concerned. The fact that the GP was not subsequently contacted may have been because her instructions were misunderstood or that there was little knowledge of the NHS or, indeed, possibly no one was able to make a phone call in English.

In a large number of cases professionals used family members to interpret. There were several difficult cases where children were used inappropriately to interpret intimate, personal or social details of the mother, and, therefore, vital information was withheld. The report makes a general recommendation about the use of interpreters. Midwives should pro-actively raise this issue with their trust managers if they are concerned.

Cultural issues also affect other groups. The report also shows that a disproportionate number of women from the traditional travelling community were likely to die.

In relation to caring for women from other cultures, midwives and other health professionals should:

- develop a greater awareness of different cultural needs
- request the use of interpreters and/or link workers from within their own organizations

- be at the forefront of developing flexible services for women who are unable, for whatever reason, to regularly attend clinic-based antenatal services.

All healthcare professionals should consider whether there are unrecognized but inherent racial prejudices within their own organizations, in terms of providing an equal service to all service users.

Domestic violence

Midwives are increasingly recognizing the impact of domestic violence on the physical and mental well-being of mothers and their families. The Department of Health and The Royal College of Midwives have produced guidelines for the detection and management of domestic violence,[12, 13] as have a number of other professional organizations. Current evidence suggests that domestic violence often starts or intensifies during pregnancy. Midwives, therefore, need to be constantly aware of the possibility, watching for the signs and symptoms suggestive of domestic violence that are discussed in depth in Chapter 16 of the current report.[6]

Twelve per cent of the women whose deaths were investigated in the last report self-reported a history of domestic violence to a healthcare professional. Many women do not admit to being victims of domestic violence due to shame or the fear of reprisal, but may do so if questioned in a sensitive manner. From the information from this enquiry, it appeared that no women had been routinely asked if they had suffered from violence as part of the social history taken at booking, so the figure of 12% is likely to be an underestimate of the prevalence of violence amongst this group of women.

Domestic violence is a difficult issue for healthcare professionals. Many may feel that by opening up the question they may be presented with a situation that they do not know how to deal with and appear to be offering the woman more support and advice than they believe they can provide. Some midwives will also have experienced violence against themselves. For these reasons it is important that not only are health professionals, including midwives, trained to understand the importance of confronting these issues, but that they are also supported by a local network of agencies to whom the woman can be referred for specialized help.

All women, whether or not they admit to suffering domestic violence, should have access to information about local services, including the local Women's Aid Help Line, Refuge and the Police

Community Safety Unit. Midwives should have available a 24-hour help-line number that they can give to women at risk of domestic violence. Midwives should consider whether all women should be given this number as part of routine practice.

Obesity

Obesity is a risk factor for maternal morbidity and mortality for a number of conditions including thromboembolism and diabetes. Many mothers who died in this triennium were classified as obese, although, as there has been a tendency not to weigh mothers routinely in pregnancy, the precise body weights were not always available. All mothers should have their body mass index (BMI) calculated at booking as part of the full risk assessment. Further, they should be offered advice about sensible weight reduction, including diet and exercise, and referral to a dietician where appropriate. BMI is defined as the weight (kg) divided by the square of height (m^2). An adult BMI greater than 30 would be classified as obese. Midwives should inform mothers who are obese about how to recognize early warning signs of complications. Midwives are also well placed to give advice on healthy eating, diet and exercise.

Professional accountability and responsibility, including advocacy

Midwives must reflect and develop their practice, and play an active role in challenging the organizational structure and culture in which they work, to agree policies that reflect the recommendations in this report. The midwife is accountable for the care she/he delivers, and should act as an advocate for women, providing a high standard of care in accordance with midwives' rules and code of practice, and guidelines for professional practice.

Advocacy

Despite excellent care for many women, some midwives appeared to miss the opportunity to question the decisions made by other professionals and act as an advocate for the women in their care. The report gives examples of circumstances where midwives failed to challenge the decisions made by GPs or junior medical staff despite having major concerns. In addition, in a few cases, the midwife co-ordinating the delivery suite did not support the midwives' concerns in that she did not summon senior medical assistance.

Midwives should feel confident to challenge areas of medical practice in a proactive manner if they are concerned, and should have the ability to refer women they are directly concerned about to hospital services. Midwives should also be prepared to decline taking responsibility for high-risk cases where the involvement of a consultant or senior obstetrician is essential, and the reasons for this should be explained to the woman and to the obstetrician.

Inappropriate responsibility for care

A small number of women who had features identifying them as high risk at the booking appointment, received shared care suitable only for low-risk women. In these cases the previous obstetric history did not appear to be part of the planning process when the care was being considered for the current pregnancy. Consultant obstetricians and midwives should be aware of the booking history prior to planning the most appropriate antenatal care. The GP booking letter is a referral mechanism and should not be relied upon to provide all the information necessary to plan antenatal care.

With the growing importance of midwifery-led care, it is vital that midwives undertake a full needs assessment at the booking visit in order to identify women whose past or current medical history may make them unsuitable for this type of care, and that these women be referred for more appropriate care. Similarly, midwives should be prepared to decline taking responsibility for high-risk cases as explained above in the section on Advocacy.

Risk assessment

The crucial role of the midwife is to perform an ongoing risk assessment of the woman from booking and then at each point of contact through the antenatal and intrapartum periods to the postnatal period. At booking, this risk assessment includes a detailed review of the woman's personal and family obstetric and medical history, with particular reference to significant risk factors, such as thromboembolism and mental illness. Appropriate action should be taken when any deviations from the normal are noted.

The importance of risk assessment at each contact is illustrated by several cases of pre-eclampsia in the latest report that may have gone undetected for some time. This may have been due to the woman being seen without a urine specimen being checked, and emphasizes the need for urinalysis at each antenatal contact after 20 weeks of pregnancy.

Midwives will wish to be aware of several new findings from this enquiry when undertaking risk assessments at booking and in the antenatal period.

Major psychiatric illness

As previously discussed, suicide is the leading cause of maternal death. Chapter 11 of the latest report, Psychiatric causes of death,[6] contains valuable new information and recommendations, many of which are particularly relevant to the provision of midwifery care.

Of great importance is the risk of recurrence in women with a past history of a previous severe postnatal depression or puerperal psychosis, or of a non-pregnancy-related condition such as bipolar illness, schizophrenia or obsessional compulsive disorder. Women with a past history of severe mental illness, be it puerperal or non-puerperal, face a risk of a recurrence of between 1 in 2 and 1 in 3 following delivery. The risk of recurrence is at its greatest in the first 30 days postpartum. Typically, these illnesses are of rapid onset, escalation of severity and of similar presentation and timing to previous puerperal episodes. This is why the recommendation made in the last report that 'a relatively simple procedure should be instituted in every antenatal clinic to identify women at risk of post-natal psychiatric illness and/or self harm' is, and will continue to be, repeated.

In a large percentage of cases clear psychiatric risk factors were present but were not ascertained. Staff, including midwives, often underestimated symptoms of depression or psychosis. For women with a past history of severe mental illness, clear multidisciplinary planning should take place because of the risk of recurrence. This should include referral pathways and criteria for triggering such a referral. There should be a low threshold for seeking intervention where there is a previous personal or family history of mental illness.

The midwife is well placed to identify women at greatest risk of psychiatric illness. This will involve the detection of risk factors at booking, such as a past history of psychosis or depression, whether postnatal or not. The midwife must also be vigilant in looking for signs and symptoms of psychiatric disease developing during pregnancy and the postnatal period. Half of all women who died from psychiatric illness in the postnatal period had a previous history of mental illness. Many of these women appeared to have good social support, but, frequently, the professionals underestimated the severity of acute presentations.

It is clear that the risk assessment for many of these women was cursory, and a relevant history was noted as postnatal depression

(PND) without any further enquiry. The women who died suffered from major psychiatric illnesses, not PND. The term 'PND' should only be used to describe a non-psychotic depressive illness of mild-to-moderate severity with its onset following delivery. It should not be used as a generic term to describe other mental illnesses. In this enquiry the use of the acronym 'PND' to describe cases of very severe illness complicating previous childbirth, may have led to the likely severity of the recurrence being underestimated and to missed opportunities for prevention.

If a woman reports a previous episode of psychiatric illness, it should not be dismissed as 'PND', but enquiry should be made about the severity of the illness, its clinical presentation, the treatment required and the timing of its onset. Most women who have experienced a previous serious postpartum illness will be concerned about future recurrence. Midwives, obstetricians, GPs and psychiatrists must know about the high risk of recurrence, and must know that women with early-onset conditions can quickly move from appearing to be merely anxious and depressed to being psychotic and suicidal within a few days. They also need to know that being mentally well in pregnancy does not necessarily reduce the risk of recurrence after delivery. Forewarned is forearmed and at the very least a period of skilled monitoring and management plans for early intervention could be instituted.

In nine deaths, where the past history had been recorded in the midwifery notes, it was referred to as 'PND', despite the evidence of previous severe psychiatric illness in relation to childbirth. In no case was there any evidence that the severity of the previous illness and, indeed, in-patient care had been ascertained. The use of the term 'PND' gave the impression that the illness had been less severe than it actually was and no appropriate referral to the psychiatric service or care plans had been made.

A number of cases involved women in their first pregnancy with a previous history of non-postpartum psychiatric illness. Again the risk of a recurrence or relapse after childbirth appears not to have been recognized either by their psychiatrists or by their midwives. This led to the care being re-active rather than pro-active. It seems that the professionals involved in these women's care were taken by surprise by the rapid escalation of symptom severity following the onset of the condition.

Thromboembolism

Thromboembolism remains the leading direct cause of maternal death. Risk factors for thromboembolism were present in 25 of the

31 cases of maternal death included in the last report. Thirteen women were overweight, five had had a period of bed rest, four had a family history, three had previous thromboembolism, and two had undertaken long-haul flights during pregnancy. Some had multiple risk factors. In spite of this multiplicity of risk factors, many of the mothers who died appeared to be treated as low risk. Identified risk factors need to be readily available to all health professionals in the antenatal and postnatal periods. If a woman appears to be at higher risk of thromboembolism, she requires referral for medical advice.

Midwives should be aware that pregnancy itself increases the risk of pulmonary embolism, which frequently presents with vague symptoms such as breathlessness. Thirteen women died from pulmonary embolism in the antenatal period. Of these, eight were in the first trimester of pregnancy. Of the 17 postnatal deaths, 10 followed a vaginal delivery.

Planning care for women at known risk of complications

Allied to the need for a risk assessment to be undertaken for all women, once a woman is known to be at higher risk of complications during pregnancy or delivery, a relevant multidisciplinary care plan should be agreed in conjunction with the woman. In several cases discussed in the report this had not been done, or was inadequate. This led to confusion as to what protocol to follow and the unavailability of key staff when the mother's condition suddenly deteriorated. However, even when appropriate care plans had been made, in a few cases the midwives and junior doctors failed to follow the written instructions and appeared not to appreciate the seriousness of these high-risk cases. It is crucial to have well-documented plans for women at identified higher risk.

Communication

The importance of communication between health professionals is a recurring theme in these reports, with poor communication being a contributory factor to the mother's death in a significant number of cases. In some instances communication with the woman was also poor.

Communication between health professionals

In many cases there was evidence of good communication and multidisciplinary working even though women died. In one instance a woman was diagnosed with cancer in early pregnancy and spent much of her pregnancy in hospital. An excellent summary of the midwifery care demonstrated good planning and communication, delivering a high standard of care. Extra care given by the midwives included liaison with other healthcare teams, staff and family conferences, and teaching basic parenting skills to the partner.

The midwife is frequently the professional that will identify factors placing the mother at high risk when taking a booking history. It is essential that the risks identified are communicated effectively to the health professionals best able to ensure that the most appropriate care be given.

Most midwives working in the community appeared to be comfortable in referring women to the secondary-care maternity services, but some did not appear to work in partnership within the primary-care setting and outside agencies. This was particularly evident in terms of communication with other members of the primary-healthcare team. If a referral to a GP is thought necessary it is preferable for the midwife to make direct contact with a GP rather than giving the responsibility to the woman herself.

Knowing when to refer

In specific instances some midwives appeared reluctant to refer across specialty borders to allied professionals, such as community psychiatric nurses, even when there was a serious risk of mental illness. Midwives need to feel comfortable and make more use of these horizontal, inter-specialty communications, as well as vertical, hierarchical communication pathways. This may involve overriding the decisions of other health professionals, perhaps by direct referral to other agencies such as A&E departments or consultant-led teams.

In several cases in the last enquiry, a midwife correctly diagnosed and referred women to the hospital services with diagnoses that had been missed by the GP. However, in a few other cases the midwife, despite her concerns, did not appear able to override the GP when, evidently, there was no investigation of the woman's symptoms. On the other hand, there was evidence that some midwives made appropriate and timely referrals based on excellent clinical knowledge and an index of suspicion even though the women eventually died.

The midwife is well placed to co-ordinate partnerships with other professionals and outside agencies such as social services. There were a number of cases in the report where closer communication between the midwifery/obstetric and social services, both ante-natally and postnatally, would have prevented the woman from slipping through the net and receiving little or no support for either her medical or social problems. This was particularly the case in a number of deaths from suicide, or in women who reported domestic violence.

Women with severe social problems often fail to attend for antenatal care, as with those suffering from substance abuse. A number of women who use drugs appear to default antenatal clinic attendance whilst attending the community drug service more regularly. Midwives should consider whether they should work in concert with social services or community drug teams, and, indeed, plan future services in consultation with the women most likely to use them. In Glasgow, where drug service users have been involved in planning their services, the uptake and attendance rate is high. Open access to antenatal clinics in conjunction with substance-abuse services, without the need for making appointments, may also improve antenatal attendance.

CONTINUUM OF HOLISTIC MIDWIFERY PRACTICE: A SUMMARY OF KEY RECOMMENDATIONS 1997–99

This section provides a summary of the key recommendations as they relate to planning the process and continuum of women-centred midwifery care. Specific clinical recommendations relating to individual medical conditions are contained in the full report or the midwifery summary, which can be obtained from *www.cemd.org.uk.*

Antenatal care

Midwives should be at the forefront of helping plan new models of service provision. The planning and delivery of maternity services should focus on regarding each woman as an individual person with different social, physical and emotional needs as well as any specific clinical factors that may affect her pregnancy. Her pregnancy should not be viewed in isolation from other important factors that may influence her health or that of her developing baby.

Each woman should have a flexible, individualized antenatal care plan drawn up at booking, which reflects her own circumstances and needs. This should be reviewed regularly throughout her pregnancy.

There may be many reasons why women may fail to attend clinic appointments. These women are at higher risk of maternal and fetal complications and death, and regular non-attendance should be personally and actively followed up by the midwife. If the reasons why she felt unable to seek care are ascertained through sympathetic questioning, then alternative arrangements should be made that suit the particular circumstances of the woman.

Targeting care is about developing services that are effective for all women but particularly for those women who would not normally actively seek help and advice. As part of the changes in the delivery of midwifery care it is crucial that new patterns of antenatal care are developed particularly for those women who are at the greatest risk. In some instances this may require individual antenatal care at home.

Interpreters should be provided for women who do not speak English. The use of family members, including children as interpreters, should be avoided if at all possible.

Booking

At booking, a needs and risk assessment should take place to ensure every woman has a flexible individual plan for their antenatal care, to be reviewed at each visit, which reflects their particular requirements for antenatal care.

With the growing importance of midwifery-led care, it is vital that midwives undertake a full needs assessment at the booking visit in order to identify women whose past or current medical history may make them unsuitable for this type of care, and that these women be referred for more appropriate care. Conversely, midwives should be prepared to decline taking responsibility for high-risk cases where the involvement of a consultant obstetrician is essential, and the reasons for this should be explained to the woman and to the obstetrician.

The GP booking letter is a referral mechanism and should not be relied upon to provide all the information necessary to plan antenatal care.

All mothers should have their BMI calculated at booking as part of the full risk assessment. Further, they should be offered advice about sensible weight reduction including diet and exercise, and referral to a dietician where appropriate. A past history or family history of thromboembolism should be sought and, if present, specialist advice should be obtained.

Midwives are uniquely placed to provide advice and support on healthy lifestyles including:

- diet and exercise
- smoking, alcohol and substance misuse
- safety in the home and workplace

- basic first-aid measures, especially for women with existing conditions, such as epilepsy
- the correct use of car seat belts
- air travel
- guidance on the warning signs of obstetric complications such as pre-eclampsia.

Enquiries about previous psychiatric history, its severity, care received and clinical presentation should be made routinely in a systematic and sensitive way at the antenatal booking clinic. Women who have a past history of serious psychiatric disorder, postpartum or non-postpartum, should be referred to a psychiatrist and a management plan should be formulated in light of the high risk of recurrence.

The term PND should only be used to describe a non-psychotic depressive illness of mild-to-moderate severity with its onset following delivery. It should not be used as a generic term to describe other mental illnesses. The use of the term PND in the maternity records may diminish the severity of previous illness and the high risk of recurrence. Precise details of any previous illness should be sought and recorded in line with the recommendation above.

Provided support services have been put in place, or local care pathways identified, all pregnant women should be routinely asked about domestic violence as part of their social history and should have the opportunity to discuss their pregnancy with a midwife, in privacy, without their partner present, at least once during the antenatal period.

Ongoing care

All providers of maternity services should ensure there are clear protocols and routes of referral to primary or secondary care when rapid assessment, investigation and treatment are required. This will involve close collaboration with other professionals in both primary and secondary care.

When referring a woman to a GP in primary care, midwives should make direct contact with the GP and not ask the woman or her family to do so on their behalf.

Midwives should have the ability to refer women they are directly concerned about to hospital services.

In order to increase the detection of pre-eclampsia, all mothers should have their urine tested at each antenatal contact after 20 weeks of pregnancy.

As an individual practitioner

Midwives must reflect and develop their practice and play an active role in challenging the organizational structure and culture in which they work, to agree policies that reflect the recommendations in this report.

Midwives and other health professionals who work with disadvantaged clients need to be able to understand a woman's social and cultural background, act as an advocate for women with medical staff and colleagues, overcome their own personal and social prejudices, and practice in a reflective manner.

Midwives should be prepared to decline taking responsibility for high-risk cases where the involvement of a consultant obstetrician is essential and the reasons for this should be explained to the woman and to the obstetrician.

Midwives need to utilize fully existing systems of statutory supervision to ensure continuing professional development and actively demonstrate evidence-based care.

Continuing professional development should be accepted as the responsibility of the individual practitioner as well as an employer, and knowledge and skills should be regularly updated using current research evidence.

References

1. Callagan W 2001 Strategies to reduce pregnancy-related deaths. In: Identification and review to action. Centres for Disease Control, American College of Obstetricians and Gynaecologists
2. World Health Organization 2001 Maternal mortality in 1995. Estimates developed by WHO, UNICEF and UNFPA. WHO, Geneva
3. Lewis G (ed.) In press. Beyond the numbers: reviewing maternal deaths and complications to make pregnancy safer. WHO, Geneva
4. Godber G 1976 The confidential enquiry into maternal deaths. In: A question of quality? Nuffield Provincial Hospitals Trusts and Oxford University Press, Oxford
5. Department of Health England 1954 Report of the confidential enquiry into maternal deaths 1952–1954. The Stationery Office, London
6. Royal College of Obstetricians and Gynaecologists 2001 Why mothers die. The United Kingdom Confidential Enquiries in to Maternal Deaths 1997–1999. The Royal College of Obstetricians and Gynaecologists, London
7. Mantel GD, Buchman E, Rees H, Pattinson RC 1998 Severe acute maternal morbidity: a pilot study of a definition of a near-miss. British Journal of Obstetrics and Gynaecology 105: 985–990

8. Waterstone M, Bewley S, Wolfe C 2001 Incidence and predictors of severe obstetric morbidity: case control study. British Medical Journal 322: 1089–1094

9. English National Board for Nursing, Midwifery and Health Visiting 2001 Report of the Board's Midwifery Practice Audit 1999/2000. English National Board for Nursing, Midwifery and Health Visiting, London

10. Department of Health 1999 Making a difference: strengthening the nursing, midwifery and health visiting contribution to health and healthcare. HMSO, London

11. Hart A, Lockey R, Henwood F, Pankhurst F, Hall V, Sommerville F 2001 Researching professional education addressing inequalities in health: new directions in midwifery education and practice. English National Board for Nursing, Midwifery and Health Visiting, London

12. Department of Health 2000 Domestic violence: a resource manual for health care professionals. Department of Health, London

13. Royal College of Midwives 1997 Domestic abuse in pregnancy. Position paper No. 19. Royal College of Midwives, London

Chapter 3

Antepartum stillbirths and strategies for prevention

Jason Gardosi

The 'unexplained' stillbirth remains the biggest problem for all involved in maternity care.[8]

Stillbirths are consistently the largest contributor to perinatal mortality in the UK and most other developed countries. The definition for stillbirth in the UK is described in full in Chapter 1. Figure 3.1 shows the trend of stillbirths, neonatal and infant deaths in England and Wales over the last 10 years. The stillbirth rates have fallen gradually from 5.7/1000 in 1993 to 5.3/1000 in 2001, but rose again to 5.6/1000 in 2002.

Perinatal deaths are collected by the Office of National Statistics (ONS) as well as through rapid report forms (RRFs) sent in by individual units to regional CEMACH offices. The two methods of data collection provide a useful means of cross-checking for ascertainment and validation.

CLASSIFICATION OF STILLBIRTHS

Conventionally, a three-tier classification is used, consisting of the pathophysiological classification by Wigglesworth,[1] the 'fetal and neonatal' classification[2] based on a system first described by Bound et al in 1954[3] and applied in the 1958 British Mortality Survey,[4] and

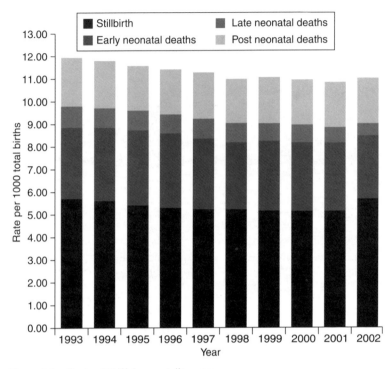

Figure 3.1 England & Wales mortality rates.
Source: Vital statistics ONS

Table 3.1 Extended Wigglesworth Classification

1. Congenital defect/malformation (lethal or severe)
2. Unexplained antepartum fetal death
3. Death from intrapartum 'asphyxia', 'anoxia' or 'trauma'
4. Immaturity
5. Infection
6. Death due to other specific causes
7. Death due to accident or non-intrapartum trauma
8. Sudden infant death, cause unknown
9. Unclassifiable

the revised Aberdeen classification[5] based on Baird and Thomson[6] first described in 1954.[7] The 'Extended Wigglesworth Classification'[8] is the one most commonly used for reporting perinatal mortality rates, and consists of 9 categories (Table 3.1).

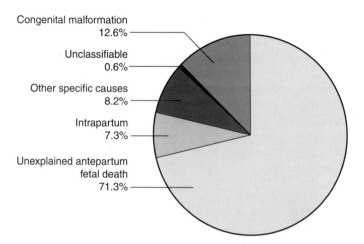

Congenital malformation
12.6%

Unclassifiable
0.6%

Other specific causes
8.2%

Intrapartum
7.3%

Unexplained antepartum
fetal death
71.3%

Figure 3.2   Stillbirths in England, Wales & Northern Ireland in 1999 by Wigglesworth classification.
Source: CESDI 8th annual report.

According to the latest published figures by the Confidential Enquiry into Stillbirths and Deaths in Infancy (CESDI),[8] the breakdown of stillbirths is as shown in Figure 3.2. 'Unexplained' stillbirths are consistently the largest category.

UNDERSTANDING STILLBIRTHS

It is a strength of the confidential enquiries that trends in mortality statistics apparent from RRFs and ONS data can be followed by targeted studies, where multiprofessional panels can look at causes and patterns of care. The panels are selected at regional level in such a way that they would not have been involved in the care of the woman or her baby. Because of this the panel members can examine the circumstances surrounding the baby's death in a confidential and objective manner. The cases are presented in an anonymous format. The confidential enquiry panel identifies any suboptimal factors surrounding care, and factors are graded using the criteria given in Table 3.2.

Several CESDI studies have looked into antepartum stillbirths over the years, trying to elucidate causes and degree of avoidability.

In the 4th CESDI Report,[9] an investigation into intrapartum deaths found that 44.9% ($n = 392$) showed evidence of suboptimal care in the antepartum period, including 89.3% ($n = 350$) that were substandard

Table 3.2   CESDI grading system

0 – No suboptimal care
I – Suboptimal care, but different management would have made no difference
II – Suboptimal care – different management MIGHT have made a difference
III – Suboptimal care – different management WOULD REASONABLY BE EXPECTED to have made a difference

Grade 2 or Grade 3, i.e. where the care could have, or was likely to have, contributed to the death.

This picture supports evidence from epidemiological studies suggesting that many intrapartum deaths have antenatal origins or factors responsible for the adverse outcome. In most cases (85.6%), the comments of panel assessors related to 'failure to recognize' or 'failure to act' on a problem. The two most common concerns were the identification and management of obstetric risk factors, and the assessment of fetal size and growth.[9] Most of the potentially avoidable deaths (Grade 2 or 3) occurred in the 'unexplained >2.5 kg' category.

Further investigation into antepartum stillbirths was carried out in the Stillbirths at Term Study (SATS) in the West Midlands (5th CESDI Report).[10] This was a case controlled study of 86 stillbirths and 170 live born controls, and excluded gestation of <37 weeks, weight of <2.5 kg, and lethal congenital anomalies. The study was underpowered, but did find two significant differences between cases and controls: an antenatal problem had been noted in twice as many cases than controls; and mothers of stillbirths were more likely to be of a non-European ethnic origin. Confidential enquiry panel assessments found that, compared with controls, cases had a significantly increased rate of antenatal care that was sub-optimal (Grade 2 or 3). Parental interviews were also undertaken but, as the authors stated, many of the questions were subject to recall bias affected by the occurrence of the stillbirths. Using the fetal/neonatal classification,[2] 67% ($n = 58$) of the fetal deaths were in the category 'unexplained >2.5 kg'. A subsequent analysis showed that, compared to controls, there was a 3.6-fold increased likelihood that the weights of stillbirths were small for gestational age.[11]

The 1:10 Enquiries in 1996/7 (6th Report)[12] focused on notified deaths between 24 weeks' gestation and up to 28 days in the postnatal period, where the fetal or neonatal weight was at least 1 kg and there was no major congenital anomaly. A total of 573 deaths were assessed, of which 422 (74%) were stillbirths, with a median gestational age of 36 weeks. The main classification groups of this cohort were unexplained (81%), followed by intrapartum-related (11%) stillbirths. Sixty per cent of stillbirths had a post mortem, which modified the diagnosis by clinical assessment in 12% of cases.

A total of 45% of stillbirths received a suboptimal care grading of 2 or 3, including 41% of those classified as 'unexplained' – suggesting that many deaths were potentially avoidable. Once again, failure to recognize a problem (50%) or failure to act appropriately (30%) were most common – rather than, for example, lack of supervision of staff or issues concerning equipment.

In the 8th Report[8] a more detailed, qualitative analysis of the results of the 1:10 enquiries was undertaken, to throw light on the suboptimal care factors that may have contributed to the adverse outcome. Although most stillbirths occur in low-risk pregnancies, in many instances where risk factors were present in early pregnancy, they were either not recognized or ignored. There were many management issues, including the failure to act on a history of 'high risk', or situations during pregnancy as they arose, lack of care plans, and inappropriate grade of staff assuming responsibility of care. In many instances, there was poor documentation and poor oral and written communication, as well as lack of information giving, e.g. on smoking cessation. Mothers also lacked an awareness of the importance of reporting decreased fetal movements, which in many instances may have been due to a failure of professionals to explain their importance. Panel assessments frequently found failures to monitor fetal growth during pregnancy, or to act appropriately when a problem was detected. Care and support after stillbirth was also often criticized – e.g. whether the appropriate investigations and tests are carried out, or whether postmortems are offered and discussed with the bereaved parents.

The review highlighted that professionals including panel members were often neither clear nor agreed on the best way to test for and monitor antenatal well-being, and there was a need for evidence based guidelines. There was also a call for easily accessible, clear protocols for maternal and fetal risk assessment during pregnancy. The predominance of cases falling into the 'unexplained' category was observed regardless of which of the three conventional classification systems was being used.

'UNEXPLAINED' STILLBIRTHS

The inadequacy of the current classification system resulting in the high category of 'unclassified' or 'unexplained' stillbirths has been apparent for some time, and the need to address the issue has been repeatedly emphasized.[8, 12] CESDI commissioned a commentary on how this problem could be addressed.[13]

The first clinical implication of the overwhelming 'unexplained' category is that it is often considered to be synonymous with 'unavoidable', which is not conducive to understanding what went wrong, not for counselling of the woman and her family, or to the development of strategies for prevention. Yet studies using CESDI data suggest a strong link between smallness for gestational age and antepartum stillbirth.[11, 14]

Epidemiological investigations into antepartum stillbirths are possible thanks to large perinatal databases, such as the one routinely collected in Sweden. Weight-for-gestational age was assessed with an adjustment for the average delay between fetal death and delivery, estimated to be 2 days.[14, 15] The analysis showed that the stillborn fetus had a high chance of having been growth restricted before demise, with an odds ratio of 5.3 if fetal growth restriction (FGR) was defined as <10th customized centile, and an odds ratio of 11.2 for FGR defined as <2.5 centile.[16] Additional evidence comes from analysis of stillbirths in Oslo, where 52% of 'unexpected' antepartum fetal deaths, which had revealed no findings on post mortem, were FGR.[17]

While fetal growth restriction is not in itself a 'cause', it is a clinically relevant condition preceding stillbirth. Clinical suspicion of slow growth can lead to referral for further investigation such as ultrasound biometry and Doppler, which are the recommended investigations.[18]

The classification system for stillbirth needs to aid our understanding of the foregoing clinical condition, in order to aid prevention.[13] A new classification has been developed which looks at the 'relevant condition at death' (ReCoDe)[19] (Table 3.3). It is based on the following principles:

- Stillbirths are distinct from neonatal deaths and warrant their own classification.
- There is hence no need for a subclassification according to gestation, as 'prematurity' is not a relevant cause or condition for stillbirths.
- There is no subclassification according to weight, but one related to fetal growth status, based on weight-for-gestation.
- The classification emphasizes what went wrong, not necessarily 'why'. Hence, more than one category can be coded.
- The hierarchy starts from conditions affecting the fetus and moves outwards, in simple anatomical categories (A–F), which are subdivided into pathophysiological conditions.
- The primary condition should be the highest on the list that is applicable to a case.

Table 3.3 Classification of stillbirths by Relevant Condition of Death

A	Fetus		
		1	Lethal congenital anomaly
		2	Infection
			2.1 Chronic – e.g. TORCH
			2.2 Acute
		3	Non-immune hydrops
		4	Iso-immunization
		5	Fetomaternal haemorrhage
		6	Twin–twin transfusion
		7	Intrapartum asphyxia
		8	Fetal growth restriction[1]
		9	Other
B	Umbilical cord		
		1	Prolapse
		2	Constricting loop or knot[2]
		3	Velamentous insertion
		4	Other
C	Placenta		
		1	Abruptio
		2	Praevia
		3	Vasa praevia
		4	Placental infarction
		5	Other placental insufficiency[3]
		6	Other
D	Amniotic fluid		
		1	Chorioamnionitis
		2	Oligohydramnios[2]
		3	Polyhydramnios[2]
		4	Other
E	Uterus		
		1	Rupture
		2	Uterine anomalies
		3	Other
F	Mother		
		1	Diabetes
		2	Thyroid diseases
		3	Essential hypertension
		4	Hypertensive diseases in pregnancy
		5	Lupus/antiphospholipid syndrome
		6	Cholestasis
		7	Drug abuse
		8	Other
G	Trauma		
		1	External
		2	Iatrogenic
	H	Unclassified	
		1	No relevant condition identified
		2	No information available

[1] Defined as <10th customized weight-for-gestation percentile (centile calculator is available at www.gestation.net/centile)
[2] If severe enough to be considered relevant
[3] Histological diagnosis

Using this method to classify 313 antepartum stillbirths in the West Midlands in 2001, it was shown that while 230 (73.5%) were 'unexplained' by the conventional Wigglesworth method, 132 of these (57.4%) fell into ReCoDe category A8 (FGR). Using ReCoDe, only 14.1% of cases had no relevant condition identified (category H1). It is apparent, therefore, that a more clinically relevant classification can shed light on the large number of 'unexplained' stillbirths, and can allow a better understanding of where the priorities need to lie for instituting strategies for prevention. The new classification has been passed to CEMACH, to be considered for adoption for all stillbirths in England and Wales.

IMPLICATIONS FOR ANTENATAL CARE

Antepartum stillbirths are the largest contributor to perinatal mortality, and many appear to be potentially avoidable. Even though this is a difficult subject matter to analyze, the CESDI project has succeeded in generating many important statements about good practice, patient safety, and inequalities in care. These are messages for health professionals as well as those responsible for developing and maintaining a system conducive to delivering optimal care.

However, CESDI reports are stacked up on our shelves and their recommendations are not necessarily accepted and implemented. Putting evidence into practice is a difficult and demanding process that has to involve many stakeholders. The panel enquiry is a valuable learning process for the professionals who take part (see Chapter 8) and can speed up implementation of key learning points, especially if they are locally relevant. However, such implementation may be patchy. In addition to maternity units and professional groups, there is a need within the new NHS landscape to also involve strategic health authorities as performance managers, and primary care trusts as commissioners of the service. It is important to raise awareness about issues that have been highlighted by CESDI and the Confidential Enquiries into Maternal Deaths (CEMD) at all levels of the health service. Often such efforts have to compete against many other NHS priorities.

There is a lack of a national strategy on stillbirths, which is even more essential now that it has become clear that a substantial proportion of deaths are associated with substandard care. There are various activities going on at local and regional level, but often with little support, and the recent severe funding cuts in the national CEMACH programme have put even these initiatives at risk. In the

West Midlands, which has one of the highest perinatal mortality rates, and the most stillbirths of any of the old CESDI regions, the health service is investing effort and resources into a co-ordinated strategy, which we hope will eventually be adopted throughout the NHS. This strategy can be summarized into five key areas and recommendations.

1 Managing high-risk pregnancy

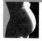 There is an urgent need to implement evidence-based protocols, multidisciplinary guidelines and care pathways.

CESDI panels have repeatedly shown that many instances of adverse outcome are the result of substandard care in cases which were 'high risk'. All professionals must be aware of risk factors based on maternal and obstetric history, and put appropriate management plans for pregnancy and delivery in place. It is also essential that vigilance is continued throughout pregnancy, as 'risk' often changes over time. Sometimes seemingly minor symptoms, for example itching, may be an important symptom of obstetric cholestasis, which may cause antenatal stillbirth.[11] Another example is the importance of maternal perception of decreased fetal movements, highlighted in the last report,[8] and the inadequacy of a CTG as primary investigation.

Within the West Midlands, increased awareness is being promoted through regular, multidisciplinary meetings and regional reviews of the evidence for best practice, which are summarized on *www.perinate. org/reviews/*. These are supplemented by locally held RAPID Workshops (Reducing Avoidable Perinatal and Infant Deaths). Where they exist, national guidelines are promoted, and in their absence, regional protocols are developed through wide consultation.

2 Fetal surveillance

 Ongoing assessment of fetal growth and well-being needs to be recognized as an essential component of antenatal care.

The strong link between adverse outcome and fetal growth failure points to the potential avoidability of many intrauterine deaths, and calls for close scrutiny of current detection and management of fetal growth restriction. Lack of detection of intrauterine growth retardation (IUGR) was also the single largest suboptimal care factor in the Euronatal Study from 10 European countries summarized in the 8th CESDI Report.[8, 20] Fetal growth needs to be assessed serially, and professionals need to be trained in fundal height measurement as the principal screening method.[21] Customized antenatal charts, which are now recommended by the Royal College of Obstetricians and Gynaecologists (RCOG),[18] have recently been implemented, and staff have been trained in 18 of the 20 maternity units in the West Midlands. Clear guidelines are established for referral and follow-up investigations, including ultrasound and Doppler.

3 Prevention and primary care

Maternity care should be led by midwives who are aware of the public health needs of their population and can work within a supportive primary-care setting.

CESDI has shown that many instances of adverse outcome occur in pregnancies that had NO risk factors from the outset. Many stillbirths present unexpectedly with the mother's arrival in the maternity unit, and remain unexplained. The need for awareness and action in response to risk factors as they develop has also been highlighted by CEMD[22] (see Chapter 2) and corresponds to the government's aims to improve patient safety.[23]

The Acheson report on health inequalities[24] describes the crucial influence of early life on subsequent mental and physical health. Policies that reduce early adverse influences on health may result in multiple benefits, not only throughout the life of that child, but also on to the next generation. The government has given a high priority to family health, with an emphasis on reducing inequality to pregnant women and young children. In response to this, there are now well-established national strategies aimed at reducing infant mortality (smoking, breast feeding, and teenage pregnancy), with further work being developed on approaches to tackling health inequalities.[25]

It is important to recognize the need to shift emphasis from an acute to a preventative model of care. Maternal and fetal surveillance needs to occur throughout each pregnancy, not just those considered 'high risk'. Follow-up should preferably be by the same health professional or small team within a primary-care setting, which encourages close involvement, joined-up working and preventative care. Antenatal visits should be regular to allow fetal growth surveillance, and allow flexibility to make best use of resources. A recently concluded pilot study in an area of high socio-economic need, the 'Bellevue Project', has demonstrated that many of these concepts can be incorporated into a model of evidence-based community midwifery care, and show significant improvement in various indicators of outcome – including Caesarean-section rates, smoking cessation, and breast feeding (the report is available on *www.perinate.org/pc-aims*).

It is apparent that midwives are well placed to really make a difference to health improvement activity in local communities.[26]

4 Pregnancy notes, information giving and good record keeping

There is a need for universal adoption of standardized maternity notes, which aids good record keeping, identification of risk factors and the development of management plans.

Poor record keeping comes up time and again as a factor associated with substandard care. Reports repeatedly call for clear identification of risk factors and management plans. The concept of hand-held pregnancy notes is widely accepted in the UK. Repeatedly, CESDI has called for the development of standardized, national notes,[10, 11] and this has been attempted through the National Maternity Record Project (NMRP) started by the RCOG in 1994. However, neither of the two versions of the NMRP notes gained acceptance and, following a review by its council, the RCOG have recently withdrawn their support from that project to open the way for other initiatives.

Last year, the Perinatal Institute concluded the development of new hand-held pregnancy notes, which are now in wide use in the West Midlands, and are currently either being considered or have already been adopted in over 30 maternity units in other regions (*www.preg.info*). They aim to address issues of patient safety and promote various CEMACH messages, such as better information giving for mothers and healthcare professionals, alerts to maternal and fetal risk factors, and the improvement of fetal-growth surveillance. Education is an important aspect of antenatal care, and by providing ample, easily understood information within the pregnancy notes, mothers and their partners are able to engage and participate in their care.

5 Denominator data on maternity and births

There is an urgent need for a routinely collected national perinatal database, which will allow the interpretation of underlying causes and trends in adverse perinatal outcome.

Stillbirths are linked to social class, deprivation and ethnicity as well as many other factors. One of the shortcomings of CEMACH's RRFs is that only 'cases' are collected. Incidence, prevalence and trends are difficult to understand without denominator data and information about the background. The high rates of stillbirths in the West Midlands, for example, are unlikely to be explained by any more substandard clinical care than in other parts of the country. Data on all pregnancies and births, as well as deaths, together with information about the baby's family background and social circumstances and the care received, will throw light on underlying causes and variations in mortality.

The need to collect denominator data from each pregnancy has often been raised at meetings about the work of CEMACH, but is a difficult task without an established IT system and without an agreed national dataset. We are in the process of introducing a web-based system for regional collection of an agreed core dataset on pregnancy, birth and neonatal care (the Maternal and Neonatal Electronic Recording System (MANNERS); *www.perinate.org/manners*). The initiative is funded by WM Specialised Services and will promote the development of safer and more cost effective neonatal networks. MANNERS will also replace our (paper based) rapid reporting system with electronic reporting of all stillbirths and neonatal deaths.

CONCLUSION

CESDI's investigations and reports over the years have many important messages for service improvement and modernization of care. They produce unique evidence which – because of the relative rarity of the event – cannot be obtained from prospective, randomized studies, yet is essential for improving the service. As concerns stillbirths, it is clear that a substantial number are potentially avoidable – including many of those that are currently classified as 'unexplained'. The causes of these avoidable deaths are manifold and concern not only the professionals, but also the care systems in which they work.

The translation of CESDI messages into practice needs to be done in a coordinated fashion, with the many stakeholders who are responsible for service delivery. However, the remit of CESDI and now CEMACH does not include implementation, and it is unclear who has the responsibility to drive this nationally. The commissioners of services have many competing priorities, and it is essential that service development in the perinatal field is pushed higher up the agenda. Hopefully, this will be aided by the National Service Framework for Maternity and Children.

References

1. Wigglesworth JS 1980 Monitoring perinatal mortality – a patho-physiological approach. Lancet 27: 684–687
2. Hey EN, LLoyd DJ, Wigglesworth JS 1986 Classifying perinatal death: fetal and neonatal factors. British Journal of Obstetrics and Gynaecology 93: 1213–1223
3. Bound JP 1956 Classification and causes of perinatal mortality. British Medical Journal ii: 1191–1196, 1260–1265
4. Butler NR 1963 Perinatal mortality: the first report of the 1958 British Perinatal Mortality Survey. E&S Livingstone Ltd, Edinburgh
5. Cole SKHE, Thomson AM 1986 Classifying perinatal death: an obstetric approach. British Journal of Obstetrics and Gynaecology 93: 1204–1212
6. Baird D, Thomson AM 1969 The survey perinatal deaths reclassified by special clinico-pathological assessment. In: Butler NR, Alberman ED (eds) Perinatal problems. E&S Livingstone Ltd, Edinburgh
7. Baird DWJ, Thomson AM 1954 The causes and prevention of stillbirths and first week deaths. Journal of Obstetrics and Gynaecology of the British Empire 61: 433–448
8. Maternal and Child Health Research Consortium 2001 CESDI 8th annual report. Department of Health, London
9. Maternal and Child Health Research Consortium 1997 CESDI 4th annual report. Department of Health, London
10. Maternal and Child Health Research Consortium 1998 CESDI 5th annual report. Department of Health, London
11. Gardosi J, Francis A, Settatree R 1999 Association between fetal growth restriction and unexplained stillbirth at term. American Journal of Obstetrics and Gynecology 180: S157
12. Maternal and Child Health Research Consortium 1999 CESDI 6th annual report. Department of Health, London
13. Gardosi J 2001 Clinical implications of 'unexplained' stillbirths. In: Confidential Enquiry into Stillbirths and Deaths in Infancy. CESDI 8th annual report. Maternal and Child Health Consortium, London, Chapter 3.4, pp 40–47
14. Gardosi J, Mul T, Mongelli M, Fagan D 1998 Analysis of birthweight and gestational age in antepartum stillbirths. British Journal of Obstetrics and Gynaecology 105: 524–530
15. Genest DR, Williams MA, Greene MF 1992 Estimating the time of death in stillborn fetuses: I. Histologic evaluation of fetal organs; an autopsy study of 150 stillborns. Obstetrics and Gynecology 80: 575–584
16. Clausson B, Gardosi J, Francis A, Cnattingius S 2001 Perinatal outcome in SGA births defined by customised versus population-based birthweight standards. British Journal of Obstetrics and Gynaecology 108: 830–834
17. Froen JF, Gardosi J, Thurmann A, Francis A, Stray-Pedersen B In press Restricted fetal growth in sudden intrauterine unexplained death. Acta Obstetrica & Gynecologica Scandinavia

18. Royal College of Obstetricians and Gynaecologists 2002 The investigation and management of the small-for-gestational age fetus. RCOG Green Top Guideline No. 31 *www.rcog.org.uk/resources/Public/Small_Gest_Age_Fetus_No31.pdf*

19. West Midlands Perinatal Institute 2001 ReCoDe – stillbirth classification system of the relevant condition at death. *www.wmpi.net/pnm/recode.htm*

20. Richardus JH, Wilco C, Graafmans et al. 2002 Differences in perinatal mortality and suboptimal care between ten European regions: results of an international audit. British Journal of Obstetrics and Gynaecology 110: 97–105

21. Gardosi J, Francis A 1999 Controlled trial of fundal height measurement plotted on customised antenatal growth charts. British Journal of Obstetrics and Gynaecology 106: 309–317

22. Lewis G, Drife J (eds) 2001 Why mothers die 1997–1999, the fifth report of the confidential enquiries into maternal deaths in the United Kingdom. Royal College of Obstetricians and Gynaecologists Press, London

23. Building a safer NHS for patients *www.doh.gov.uk/buildsafenhs/*

24. The Independent Inquiry into Inequalities in Health 1998 Report of the independent inquiry into inequalities in health. The Stationery Office, London *www.doh.gov.uk/healthinequalities/*

25. Department of Health 2002 Tackling health inequalities, summary of the cross cutting review. Department of Health Publications, London

26. Edwards G, Gordon U, Atherton J In press Developing the midwifery contribution to public health. British Journal of Midwifery

Chapter **4**

Intrapartum-related deaths

Mary Sidebotham

It is only by knowing where we came from, and assessing where we are now, that we can see how far we have travelled.

INTRODUCTION

Birth is a journey that some would describe as the most hazardous voyage one will ever be required to undertake. It is certain that death will ultimately follow birth for all, but the challenge to professionals supporting a woman throughout her reproductive years is to promote safe motherhood. Safe motherhood is a stated aim of the World Health Organization (WHO)[1] and is supported by the former Confidential Enquiry into Maternal Deaths (CEMD) and Confidential Enquiry into Stillbirths and Deaths in Infancy (CESDI). It is now encompassed into the role of CEMACH and is fully supported by all professional and lay organizations supporting childbirth.

The concept of safe motherhood implies the measurable outcome of a healthy mother and infant, both well equipped to achieve optimal health throughout life. This aim is achievable with careful preparation, monitoring and assessment of the mother and fetus both before and during pregnancy, labour and delivery. In order to achieve these aims we must be certain that all of the models of care provided for childbearing women are designed to optimize the health of mother and baby.

The structure of all models of care should be based on the concept that birth is a normal physiological process and women should be supported through this process. Any hazards or potential blocks that may deter the safe passage of the infant through the process of birth, should be managed, and where appropriate removed. Where assistance along the route is required by the mother or the fetus, it should be timely, apt and carried out by an appropriately trained practitioner in accordance with recognized evidence-based standards of good practice. All professionals supporting a woman through pregnancy and birth should have immediate access to the resources, training and expertise required to support the safe passage of the fetus wherever that birth is taking place.

As discussed in Chapter 1, one of the measures currently being used to assess whether or not these basic principles are being met, is analysis at local, national and international level of the perinatal mortality rate. It is the examination of crude perinatal mortality rates that has influenced much of the work undertaken by CESDI, and examination of factors contributing to perinatal loss has determined the work programme for the confidential enquiries.

The overall aim of CESDI was 'to improve understanding how the risks of death in late fetal life and infancy, from 20 weeks of pregnancy to one year after birth may be reduced.'[2] However, has that aim been achieved? This chapter will look specifically at the impact of the confidential enquiry programme on reducing intrapartum-related deaths.

The following topics will be discussed to assist the reader in relating theory to practice and aid in the understanding of how the confidential enquiry programme has added to the structure of safe modern maternity services:

- The background to the enquiry programme and the wider work programme.
- Intrapartum-related deaths that are published in the 4th annual CESDI report.[3]

- The CESDI/CEMD contribution to the NHS modernization agenda national policy and labour ward guidelines.
- Examples of partnership working and collaboration to identify and reduce risk.
- Midwifery supervision. The contribution to safe modern maternity services.
- Future challenges.

BACKGROUND TO THE ENQUIRY PROGRAMME AND THE WIDER WORK PROGRAMME

One of the major strengths of the CESDI work programme is the independent peer review of carefully selected cases and controls. The confidential enquiry programme has produced recommendations for practice that are now a fundamental feature of labour ward guidelines throughout the country. Those recommendations are endorsed by the Clinical Negligence Scheme for Trust (CNST) and have resulted in collaborative working by the major professional organizations to produce information for professionals on how to best take those recommendations forward into practice.[4] It is vital, therefore, that the confidential enquiry programme is timely, relevant and focussed on an area where improvements in care could reasonably be anticipated.

The basic data used by CESDI to inform the confidential enquiry programme since its launch is that contained within the rapid report form (RRF), which is described in Chapter 1.

When the local CEMACH coordinator completes the RRF, each death is classified identifying the maternal and fetal factors associated with the death. A further classification, the Wigglesworth classification, is applied to note the more general factors associated with the death. These classifications can be found in any of the CESDI reports which can be downloaded from the CEMACH web site *www. cemach.org.uk*. The information collected on the RRF has been used within perinatal surveys on a regional basis, but it is the wider national analysis that has enabled trends in perinatal and infant loss to be demonstrated. It is through this wider analysis of larger numbers that CESDI have been able to demonstrate the areas where enquiries should be focussed. As the data collection is continuous CESDI have also been able to demonstrate any trends in classification data following publication of recommendations. This is especially significant for intrapartum related deaths as the 8th CESDI report[5] demonstrated clear evidence that improvements have been made in reducing intrapartum-related deaths which accounted 0.95 deaths per 1000 live births in 1994, but fell to 0.62 per 1000 in 1999.[6] The Wigglesworth classification describes an intrapartum death as:

Death from intrapartum 'asphyxia', 'anoxia' or 'trauma': This category covers any baby who would have survived but for some catastrophe occurring during labour. These babies will tend to be normally formed, stillborn or with poor Apgar scores, possible meconium aspiration or evidence of acidosis. Very premature infants (those less than 24 weeks gestation) may be asphyxiated at birth, but should not be entered in this category as a rule. (Wigglesworth classification 3)

INTRAPARTUM-RELATED DEATHS: CESDI 4TH ANNUAL REPORT

A total of 873 intrapartum-related deaths of babies born in 1994 and 1995 were subjected to confidential panel review. These babies were all over 1000 g and had no life-threatening abnormalities. The panels were selected in a similar manner to the panels described in Chapters 1 and 3, and consisted of clinicians from different disciplines. These included as a minimum an obstetrician, paediatrician, midwife, pathologist and a GP. Other professionals were included where appropriate. Each case was discussed in detail and any evidence of suboptimal care was recorded. The panel graded the severity of the suboptimal care using the following criteria:

- 0 – No suboptimal care
- I – Suboptimal care, but different management would have made no difference
- II – Suboptimal care, but different management MIGHT have made a difference
- III – Different management WOULD REASONABLY BE EXPECTED to have made a difference.

The 4th annual CESDI report concluded that of the 873 intrapartum-related deaths subjected to confidential peer review, 78% ($n = 681$) had suboptimal factors surrounding care. In 25% ($n = 219$) it was thought that different care might have made a difference to the outcome, but in 53% ($n = 462$) it was felt by the panels that different care would be reasonably expected to have made a difference to outcome. These deaths were thought to be the potentially avoidable deaths. Within all CESDI/CEMD reports where intrapartum events have been assessed for contributory factors to that death, common themes have emerged. These are:

- lack of senior involvement in the management of cases
- poor/inappropriate communication
- poor record keeping
- failure to recognize a problem
- failure to act on a problem
- misinterpretation of results
- lack of resources and or equipment.

The comments supporting the overall assessment fell within the broad categories described above and each case may have been assessed to show one or all factors.

ENQUIRY THEMES EVIDENT WHERE CARE WAS SUBOPTIMAL

There were several specific areas of suboptimal care that have implications for midwifery practice and warrant further discussion.

Inefficient monitoring of fetal well-being in labour

Examples of this included:

- poor-quality cardiotocograph (CTG) recording with no attempt to perform an ultrasound scan to check for presence of a fetal heart
- failure to attach a fetal scalp electrode (FSE) where external monitoring was of poor quality
- attachment of an FSE where the quality of an external trace was good, rather than recourse to further action based on the interpretation of the CTG
- misinterpretation of abnormal CTG
- failure to take appropriate action in the presence of an abnormal CTG
- failure to refer to senior obstetrician/midwife in the presence of CTG abnormality
- failure to perform fetal blood sampling (FBS)
- inappropriate action in response to FBS results
- there were cases highlighting differences of opinion on interpretation of CTG, or the need for FBS between professionals. In these cases there was lack of accountability demonstrated, as

the person with the valid concern often did not seek a second opinion.

Lack of risk recognition and categorization; inadequate case management and organizational deficiencies

Examples included:

- failure to recognize risk factors and plan care accordingly
- lack of senior obstetric input in the management of cases.

Example 1

Panels critisized consultants for not attending personally where this was indicated, and/or giving advice that was ambiguous or for giving advice that delayed effective action.

- Failure to recognize a problem and seek further advice
- Lack of resources
- On some occasions where competent assistance was technically available, they were occupied elsewhere with no back-up procedures evident.

Example 2

The obstetric SHO was left without support due to the registrar being busy in theatre, to attempt ventouse (failed), in a patient with obstructed labour who was not at full dilatation ... a junior doctor should not be put in this position.

- Record keeping errors were cited as a major contributing factor to failures in communication
- Organizational deficiencies were criticized where there was no evidence of an effective procedure in place to deal with a deviation from the norm.

Example 3

There is an impression in the notes that the organization of equipment and staff was not as such to mount an effective response promptly when problems arose ... There was a panel consensus that the ultimate loss of this baby resulted from a gradual descent into an almost irretrievable position.

Lack of organization and poor communication at transfer of care from one professional to another. This was apparent both at shift handover or where care was transferred for one unit to another.

Labour management prior to delivery

Induction of labour was highlighted as a recurring theme associated with poor outcome, as was the augmentation of labour with syntocinon. There were concerns regarding the use of prostaglandin and syntocinon related to the inadequacy of fetal monitoring throughout the process.

> **Example 4**
>
> *Attendants often seemed to ignore the implication that induction was performed on the basis of some increased risk and continued to manage induced labour as though it were low risk.*
>
> Regardless of whether labour was spontaneous or induced there were examples of mismanagement of poor progress in labour ranging from misuse of syntocinon in the presence of severe fetal distress, to lack of awareness of clinical signs of impending uterine rupture.

Management of delivery

The most frequently cited factor was the delay in decision making at all stages in the process, up to and including performing Caesarean section. Reasons varied and included inappropriate waiting for results, failure to communicate the urgency of the situation to the multi-disciplinary team and failure to recognize the gravity of a problem.

Negative comments surrounding the actual conduct of delivery were primarily directed at attempts to perform vaginal delivery. The recurring theme throughout the assessment of conduct of delivery was the assumed inexperience of the accoucher. This was shown to be a significant factor when assessing cases where the primary reason for fetal loss was assessed by the panel to be due to inadequate management of breech delivery or shoulder dystocia, and the inappropriate attempts by junior staff to perform difficult ventouse or forceps deliveries unsupervised.

Neonatal resuscitation

Within the 873 intrapartum-related deaths presented in the 4th CESDI report, there were 375 neonatal deaths that were categorized as fulfilling the Wigglesworth 3 criteria for intrapartum-related deaths. The overall grade made by assessors was 2 or 3 in 81% of these deaths ($n = 303$). Of these, it was assessed that in 22% of cases ($n = 81$) suboptimal post-delivery care may have possibly or probably contributed to the death of the baby.

Whilst it can be inferred in some cases that any attempt to resuscitate the baby would have been unsuccessful due to mismanagement prior to delivery, there were inadequacies and errors in management that assessors felt directly contributed to the baby's death in 81 cases. The themes follow the same trend observed in all of the confidential enquiries:

- Lack of organization and preparation
- Failure to recognize the problem
- Failure to respond appropriately
- Failures in communication
- Lack of clinical expertise/inadequate training
- Lack of resources.

The following case effectively demonstrates the cascade effect of these recurring themes on poor outcome.

Example 5

Resuscitation at birth was not vigorous enough. Baby described as shocked and cyanosed at 10 minutes but not intubated until 30 minutes after birth. No attempt was made to take blood pressure until flying squad arrived. No attempt to remove meconium at time of intubation. Low blood sugar not corrected. No record of blood gas results.

The initial good heart rate and tone suggest, however, that the hypoxia at birth may not have been profound. Some of the damage may, therefore, have occurred post delivery due to hypotension and meconium aspiration compounded by inadequate ventilation. It is possible that some of this damage could have been prevented by more vigorous resuscitation efforts immediately after post delivery.

4TH CESDI REPORT RECOMMENDATIONS: ENQUIRY TO ACTION

Following multidisciplinary peer review of these cases, it was evident that major changes in practice and policy were required. The report authors concluded that the following recommendations be taken on board and acted upon without delay:

- Training, assessment, supervision and practice of obstetricians and midwives of all grades needs to be critically appraised by their parent bodies.

- The Royal Colleges and other institutions responsible for teaching and accreditation should examine how the levels of practical competence of professionals of all grades, caring for women in labour and for babies, are achieved and maintained.

- The quality of maternity records needs to be improved to enable clear identification of risk factors and documentation of management plans for these during both antepartum and intrapartum periods. This would be facilitated by a well-designed universally used national maternity record.

- The establishment of a multidisciplinary initiative is needed to develop guidelines covering all aspects of fetal assessment before and especially during labour. They should cover training and assessment for all professionals using CTGs. Training should include interpretation, management options and lines of communication when abnormality is detected.

Other areas where multidisciplinary guidelines were deemed necessary included:

- professionals' responsibility for decision making when problems are identified
- inter-professional communication and responsibility for handover or sharing of care arrangements
- induction and augmentation of labour
- conduct of operative deliveries
- neonatal resuscitation.

Within the intrapartum-related deaths there were specific areas of practice that warranted further detailed peer review, and one of the recommendations of the 4th report was that focus groups be developed to 'provide specific recommendations for some uncommonly encountered but highly contributory causes of stillbirth and neonatal death'. The reports from the focus groups that reviewed specific areas of practice were published in the 5th and 6th reports[6,7] and are examined in detail in Chapter 6, but the overarching conclusion remains the same.

Peer review of 873 intrapartum deaths occurring in 1994 suggested that 681 babies might not have died with different care. However, the challenge is how to ensure that the recommendations made by CESDI based on the findings of confidential enquires become enshrined in practice.

Uptake of the 4th report recommendations

Setting the scene

The government white paper *The New NHS; Modern and Dependable*[8] was published in 1997 introducing the government's vision of review and modernization of the NHS. The associated publication *A First Class Service; Quality in the NHS*[9] introduced the proposed structure to take that vision of a safe modern dependable NHS forward. The major themes running through the proposed modernization agenda were:

- promoting safety
- reducing risk
- improving quality.

At the same time there was a growing media interest in high-profile cases involving clinical issues, and a growing awareness at professional and public level of the need for transparency and account-ability within the structure, delivery and management of the NHS. The public needed reassurance that services were safe and the staff working within them were knowledgeable, competent and subject to professional regulation. The NHS and the professionals working within it had to be seen to be accountable.

It was within this culture of a government agenda committed to improvement that the recommendations of the 4th CESDI report and those following on from focus group work were set.

The framework for the new NHS outlined within the *First Class Service* publication provided the solutions on a national scale that would provide a forum to ensure that the recommendations would be moved into practice to reduce risk.

NATIONAL INSTITUTE OF CLINICAL EXCELLENCE

The National Institute of Clinical Excellence (NICE) was established as a special health authority for England and Wales in April 1999. Its role is to provide patients, health professionals and the public with authori-tative, robust and reliable guidance on current best practice.[10] The clinical guideline programme established by NICE has had a signifi-cant impact on maternity services, and the confidential enquiry pro-grammes have informed the committees involved in the structuring of the national evidence-based guidelines that are in use in the UK and beyond. There are now clear guidelines available advising on manage-ment of induction of labour and the use of electronic fetal monitoring in labour.[11] Recommendations for basic minimum standards of training have been produced for the use of electronic fetal monitoring, which, if widely implemented, should help address the biggest area of error and concern surrounding the intrapartum-related death enquiry: 'the misuse and misinterpretations of CTGs before and during labour'.

Part of the wider-reaching work of NICE is the production of the National Service Frameworks (NSF). The emerging findings from the Children's National Service Framework[12] will further guide maternity and neonatal services to help ensure that the good practice achieved through improved guidelines and training packages is further built upon and used to support safe equitable care for all. The fivefold increased risk of stillbirth and intrapartum-related neonatal death in women with diabetes[13-15] was confirmed through RRF notifications to CESDI, and has informed the work of the diabetes NSF. The CEMACH diabetes programme will, ultimately, produce recommendations to further reduce the risk of death from intrapartum-related events of babies whose mothers have diabetes.

CLINICAL GOVERNANCE

The publication and enactment of *A First Class Service; Quality in the NHS* placed a statutory duty on the chief executive of each NHS trust to ensure the quality of services within the trust. Whilst most units prior to 1999 had systems in place to monitor service provision through an audit programme, in many cases this was done in an ad hoc manner, and the audit and quality improvement budget often bowed to the competing pressures for clinical service provision. The vesting of responsibility for quality with the chief executive ensured this would not happen. From April 1st 1999 each trust has had to demonstrate a clinical governance agenda that promoted a change in organizational culture in a systematic and demonstrative way moving away from a culture of blame to one of learning. Clinical governance promotes sharing of practice and the pursuit of evidence-based medicine. There is a requirement for each professional within an organization to recognize their own contribution to the patient's journey through services. Clinical governance promotes the concept of personal accountability. Each individual must work collaboratively within a multidisciplinary team to promote evidence-based practice, ensure that standards are met and poor practice is challenged. It is the ultimate responsibility of the chief executive to ensure that systems are in place to ensure that this happens.

There is a requirement within the governance agenda to ensure full commitment to the principle of life-long learning and continual professional development.

The value of the confidential enquiry programme in promoting this culture was well recognized and the governance agenda places a direct responsibility upon all trusts to commit fully to the national confidential enquiry programme.

Through the clinical governance agenda trusts are obliged to have in place clear reporting systems to identify and learn from adverse incidents. There must be a real and demonstrable ability within trusts to learn from experience, and avoid the lessons highlighted by failure.[16] The recently published report *An Organisation with a Memory*,[17] highlighted the same recurrent theme seen within the confidential enquiry programme.

> *Failures often have a familiar ring, displaying strong similarities to incidents which have occurred before, and in some cases almost exactly replicating them. Many could be avoided if only the lessons of experience were properly learned.*[18]

Clinical incident reporting systems, designed to manage risk, promote accountability and ensure practice changes as a result of incident reporting should be present in all organizations. All staff should be committed to the no-blame culture, crucial to ensure that these systems are used effectively by all.

The governance agenda requires each trust to show good systems are in place to monitor performance and identify and rectify training needs. In order to improve and move on from the situation in 1997, it was evident that there needed to be a substantial investment in training. Whilst NICE have produced the guidelines, and the Royal Colleges have sought the evidence, the professional organizations have developed packages and materials and provided training designed to meet the needs of professionals who needed to update their knowledge. It is through the governance agenda, however, that trusts have shown their commitment to training, which can only contribute to a better and safer service, delivered by a competent work force.

CLINICAL NEGLIGENCE SCHEME FOR TRUSTS

The Clinical Negligence Scheme for Trusts (CNST) was established in 1994 to provide a means for NHS trusts to fund the cost of clinical negligence litigation and to encourage effective management of claims and risk. The National Health Service Litigation Authority (NHSLA), a special health authority, administers the scheme. Membership is voluntary and open to all NHS and primary-care trusts in the country. Funding for the scheme is on a pay as you go, non-profit making basis. Actuaries appointed by the NHSLA calculate from the data available to them, the predicted amount expected to be paid in respect of damages, costs and other expenses in the ensuing financial year. This amount is then apportioned between the members of the scheme. Individual trust contributions are based on a range of pre set criteria. The amount paid into the scheme will be less for those organizations that can demonstrate that effective measures have been put into place to reduce the incidence of adverse incidents which could potentially lead to a claim against the organization for damages.[18] The more cynical person may feel that the sole purpose of CNST is to reduce the amount of money paid out to patients following adverse outcomes related to clinical negligence. However, the fact remains that as a government-funded organization CNST is committed first and foremost to patient safety. The actual aim, therefore, of CNST is to contribute to the governance agenda within trusts, and to promote quality and safe equitable standards of care for all patients using NHS services. A reduction in litigation and consequential costs is a welcome result, but it is not the main impetus.

CNST provide indemnity to trusts against claims for medical negligence and the level of indemnity provided is guided by the quality of the service when measured against evidence-based standards provided for the users of that service.

CNST are guided by the growing evidence base in obstetric, midwifery and neonatal care, much of which has been informed by the confidential enquiry programme, to produce standards that will promote choice, safety and remove the risk as far as is possible of adverse incident and outcome. Whilst the standards produced are generic and apply to a whole trust, the fact remains that maternity services in England account for a significant proportion of the number and costs of claims made to NHSLA each year. In response to this, specific risk management standards exclusively aimed at maternity services have been produced.[19] This initiative has been developed in response to requests from within maternity services to help to develop systems to improve outcomes and reduce risk. The development of specific evidence-based maternity standards will also support the objective set by *An Organisation with a Memory* to reduce the risk in obstetrics by 25% by 2005. All trusts providing maternity services will now be assessed specifically against the maternity standards with the rest of the trust undergoing a separate assessment for their remaining services against the existing CNST risk-management standards. It is important though to realize that a maternity service cannot operate in isolation from the trust or, indeed, from primary care. It is essential, therefore, that close and visible links are maintained. The call for improved evidence of collaboration across disciplines has been highlighted on numerous occasions with the confidential enquiry reports, and it is essential through the CNST assessment process to show the value and importance of those close links.

COLLABORATIVE WORKING

On February 1st 1999 the document *Towards Safer Childbirth: Minimum Standards for The Organisation Of Labour Wards*[4] was jointly launched by the RCM and RCOG. The document and guidelines represent the findings of the joint working party established in direct response to concerns raised within the 4th and 5th CESDI reports and also the 1994–96 triennial CEMD report.[20] The guidelines presented and endorsed by the colleges should form the basis of good working practice on every unit providing intrapartum care.

Whilst looking at those guidelines now one may find it difficult to imagine a time when such levels of service provision did not exist, but the challenge now is to ensure that those guidelines are not just recorded and logged within intranet providers and carefully thumbed folders on delivery suites, but that they are real, visible in practice and making a difference.

For example, minimum 40-hour consultant supervision, should mean that the consultant is available on the labour ward, supporting the junior trainees. The presence should be visibly teaching and sharing clinical expertise. In order to be effective and change outcomes senior staff should be actively involved in the daily work of the delivery unit. Practice may stagnate and possibly worsen in units where there is an assumption of 40-hour consultant supervision, which in reality is a 40-hour consultant availability.

The multidisciplinary labour ward forum should be an interactive forum where good practice is applauded, and poor or outdated practice is challenged and where necessary changed in line with the emerging evidence base. It is the purpose of the forum to ensure that the labour ward environment is constantly updated. The labour ward team, through the forum, should work together to promote practice reflection and the development of a supportive nurturing environment. The forum should be able to demonstrate reflection and a response to incidents that is evidence based and where appropriate consumer led.

Training in the interpretation of CTG and the management of obstetric emergencies should be mandatory for all staff working within intrapartum care and that training should be designed with an element to ensure that learning has taken place.

The colleges have taken the recommendation made by CESDI and CEMD very seriously and since publication of the minimum standards have maintained their commitment to collaborative working to reduce risk.

PROFESSIONAL REGULATION

The 4th CESDI report highlighted not just that 78% of intrapartum deaths had potentially avoidable factors but also that in >50% of those cases the failures in care could be directly attributed to the medical or midwifery staff involved in delivery of care. There was a growing awareness of a need to improve professional regulation whilst avoiding damaging the important links developing within the growing governance agenda between professional groups. The introduction of clinical governance alongside improvements within the structure of training has made each professional become more aware of their own professional accountability. Medical staff now have to show evidence of ongoing professional development in order to achieve accreditation. Midwives and nurses must show evidence of ongoing learning and reflection in order to meet the minimum standards set by the Nursing and Midwifery Council for post-registration education and practice (PREP). Midwives and nurses unable to demonstrate evidence of continued learning will not be able to renew their registration status and will, therefore, be unable to practice.

MIDWIFERY SUPERVISION

Midwifery supervision is enshrined within statute with a primary purpose to protect the public. Every practising midwife is required to notify her intention to practice, and should have the opportunity to discuss her practice with a supervisor of midwives. There has been a robust system in place for in excess of 100 years of regulating midwifery practice and addressing inadequacies and where necessary incompetencies through this tried and tested system. One wonders then, where was midwifery supervision and what was the reaction to the perceived inadequacies highlighted by the confidential enquiry panels following publication of the 4th report. It is possible that there was no multidisciplinary reflection and learning in 1994 as systems to support that culture were not in place. Midwives may have been seen on an individual basis by their supervisor, but systems did not support cultural learning. With the introduction of clinical governance there has been awareness raising throughout the NHS of the value of reflection. There is now visible support for assisting learning through critical incident review. Midwifery supervision has been used as an example as to how supported learning with clear objectives can support safe practice generically when looking at the system in place of supervised practice. Of the numbers of practitioners referred to the former UKCC for allegations of poor practice, very few were midwives as many incidents are reported and acted on within the statutory model of supervised practice. In the recent public consultation and review of regulation of nursing and midwifery, prior to the production of the new order governing the professions, the value of supervision was recognized and has been retained within the new order. It is the responsibility of all supervisors of midwives to support individual practitioners and ensure they are well equipped through training and resources to deliver safe evidence-based practice within any setting and this should include the work of the confidential enquiries.

The supervisor is, therefore, ideally placed to challenge practice, and should do so in all situations where guidelines are outdated or not followed. The supervisor is more often seen as the woman's advocate and should be available to listen to the woman's views as it is often from the women that we are given the best solutions to problems especially those involving lack of organization and communication.

COMMUNICATION

One of the major recommendations of the 4th report and every subsequent confidential enquiry report since has been to improve communication, particularly through improved standards of record keeping. Standards developed through midwifery supervision have been used as a basis for many of the multidisciplinary record keeping audits used by trusts to demonstrate improvements in standards of record keeping as required by CNST standards. There must be an ongoing commitment to the improvement in communication. The national maternity record has been developed and is in use within a large number of units, but it is not universal and does not, at present, cover intrapartum and postpartum care. In addition, there has been a welcome move towards the development of regional guidelines alongside the work of the national guideline committee. The introduction of national evidence-based guidelines will improve communication systems and reduce the opportunity for error, as clinicians moving through regions and units will be familiar with a nationally agreed known model. The value of using a regional or a national guideline has been demonstrated to improve care in the management of pre-eclampsia and the concept to extend the programmes should be welcomed and encouraged.

TRAINING AND DEVELOPMENT

Professional regulation and accreditation requirements are in place to ensure that all practising clinicians are aware of their personal responsibility to access training to ensure that their practice is safe. The CNST requirements alongside the clinical governance agenda places a responsibility on trusts to ensure that systems are in place to support training for all staff to enable them to deliver safe care. The messages from the enquires have been endorsed by CNST and an example of this is that all trusts are required to show robust evidence that CTG training is in place. The number of practitioners trained in neonatal life support (NLS) and advanced life support in obstetrics (ALSO) is increasing. There is a growing movement by all trusts to develop in house guidelines in response to ALSO and NLS training packages to ensure that consistency and continuity prevails thus reducing the risk of error.

FUTURE CHALLENGES

There is a growing concern both nationally and internationally about the rising Caesarean section rate. This has occurred with no observed reduction in perinatal mortality or morbidity. The concern is that maternal morbidity is increasing with no measurable benefit.[21, 22] Whilst one could understand there being a reactionary rise in operative deliveries in response to the findings of the intrapartum-related death enquiry, there is no evidence to support the rise has had an impact on reducing perinatal loss. There is an urgent need to redress this problem and turn the tide. Women and clinicians need to examine their practice and promote the concept of birth as a safe physiological process.

CONCLUSION

When the 4th CESDI report was published in 1997 there was a sense of shock within the professions and within organizations. Examination of systems took place to look for reasons why intrapartum care could have been so badly managed in so many cases. A major strength of the enquiry findings was its independence, and the impact was greater because the criticisms of care came from the caregivers themselves. The multidisciplinary peer-review aspects of the enquiry process caused people to take notice and those professionals who had been involved in the peer-review process took messages back to their individual units determined to make changes and reduce the risk of making the same mistakes.

However, individuals, no matter how committed, cannot effect organizational and cultural change alone. It was evident that a major shift was required accompanied by resources and commitment at government level to respond to and take action based on the recommendations of the 4th and subsequent CESDI reports. It is fortuitous and timely that the publication of the 4th report coincided with the publication of the government's plans to modernize the NHS.

The introduction of the clinical governance agenda, with its requirements to promote practice-based audit, and the development of stringent evidence-based guidelines, and strong risk-management and reporting systems, have provided the template to make the changes that were highlighted as essential back in 1997 and, in subsequent reports, to reduce the incidence of suboptimal care and subsequently intrapartum-related deaths. CNST requires that units provide proof of their adherence to standards, but how do we know that the person who is trained in neonatal resuscitation will be on duty and have access to the appropriate equipment at delivery? More importantly, how do we know that the people present at delivery will recognize that a baby needs resuscitation and call the appropriate personnel in time?

The questions that we must all ask ourselves are these:

- Is clinical governance and its huge commitment to quality affecting a real cultural change, or is it proving to be a paper exercise?
- Can we really measure individual performance and can we ensure that every practitioner responsible for providing intrapartum care is knowledgeable, competent and accountable?
- What course of action is open to a practitioner working within this modern and dependable NHS who is concerned that practice is unsafe and lives are at risk?

It is only if we can answer these questions confidently and know the responses will be positive that we can be sure that systems are in place to reduce the potential for suboptimal care to contribute to the intrapartum-related death of a baby in the future.

There was a statistically significant reduction in intrapartum deaths reported in 2000[21] and the challenge we all face now is to maintain and further improve that reduction. It is through measurable improvements in perinatal statistics like this that we judge our success. The improvements in quality can be assessed by the number of trusts achieving CNST level 3 and the maternity benchmark. The recently published report from CNST shows that: 'The maternity specific standards have clearly been well received by clinicians and have been endorsed by both the Royal College of Midwives and Royal College of Obstetricians and Gynaecologists. The main areas of non-compliance are the new criteria, which is encouraging, in respect of the older standards that are now being addressed. This success may demonstrate that CNST are driving change in the approach to clinical risk management, by supporting the national agenda and complementing the Department of Health, and other initiatives for safer clinical practice.'[23]

There are exciting and challenging times ahead for all providers of care within maternity and neonatal services. It is essential that the excellent work achieved by the confidential enquiry programme is maintained and extended. There is a growing concern at the numbers of midwives and doctors leaving the professions, and issues relating to pressures of work and fear of litigation cannot be ignored. Consumer expectations are rising all the time and it is essential that systems are in place to support the carers.

The government must commit the resources required to deliver the training programmes necessary to ensure equitable access to safe practice for all women. There must also be a visible commitment to recruitment and retention of midwives and doctors. Inadequate staffing levels on labour wards will have an inevitable impact on intrapartum deaths unless there is a redress, so whilst we can see clear progress has been made the journey is far from ended.[24] The major challenge though is that we keep moving forward from this point rather than slip back. On the advice of many an old midwife advising a woman in labour, we should all continue to push just a little bit harder.

References

1. World Health Organization 1994 Mother–baby package: Implementing safe motherhood in countries. WHO, Geneva
2. Maternal and Child Health Research Consortium 1995 CESDI 2nd annual report. Department of Health, London
3. Maternal and Child Health Research Consortium 1997 CESDI 4th annual report. Department of Health, London
4. The Royal College of Obstetricians and Gynaecologists and the Royal College of Midwives 1999 Towards safer childbirth: minimum standards for the organisation of labour wards. The Royal College of Obstetricians and Gynaecologists, London
5. Maternal and Child Health Research Consortium 2001 CESDI 8th annual report. Department of Health, London
6. Confidential Enquiries into Stillbirths and Deaths in Infancy 1998 CESDI 5th annual report. Maternal and Child Health Consortium, London
7. Maternal and Child Health Research Consortium 1999 CESDI 6th annual report. Department of Health, London

8. Department of Health 1997 The new NHS; modern and dependable. Department of Health, London
9. Department of Health 1998 A first class service: quality in the new NHS. Department of Health, London
10. National Prescribing Centre 2001 Implementing NICE guidance. Radcliffe Medical Press, Oxon
11. The Royal College of Obstetricians and Gynaecologists Clinical Effectiveness Support Unit 2001 The use of electronic fetal monitoring evidence based. Guideline no 8. The Royal College of Obstetricians and Gynaecologists, London
12. Department of Health 2003 Getting the right start: national service framework for children, young people and maternity services. Part 1: the NSF emerging findings consultation document. Department of Health, London
13. Hawthorne G, Irgens LM et al. 2000 Outcome of pregnancy in diabetic women in the North of England and in Norway, 1994–7. British Medical Journal 321: 730–731
14. Casson IF, Clarke CA et al. 1997 Outcomes of pregnancy in insulin dependent diabetic women: results of a five year population cohort study. British Medical Journal 315: 275–278
15. Hadden DR, McCance D et al. 1998 Ten year outcome of diabetic pregnancy in Northern Ireland: the case for centralisation. Diabetic Medicine 15(Suppl 1): S16
16. Lugon M, Secker C, Walker J 2001 Advancing clinical governance. Royal Society of Medicine Press, London
17. Department of Health 2000 An organisation with a memory. Report of an expert group on learning from adverse incidents in the NHS. The Stationery Office, London
18. National Health Service Litigation Authority 2002 Clinical risk management standards. Willis, Bristol
19. National Health Service Litigation Authority 2002 Clinical risk management standards for maternity services. Willis, Bristol
20. Department of Health 1998 Why mothers die: report on the confidential enquiries into maternal deaths in the United Kingdom, 1994–1996. Department of Health, London
21. The Royal College of Midwives 2000 The rising caesarean rate causes and effects for public health. Conference Proceedings. The Royal College of Midwives, London
22. The Royal College of Midwives 2002 The rising caesarean rate from audit to action. Conference Report. The Royal College of Midwives, London
23. National Health Service Litigation Authority 2003 Clinical risk management standards for maternity services. Report on the benchmarking of the CNST maternity standards between October 2002 to March 2003. NHSLA
24. Ashcroft B, Elstein M, Boreham N, Holm S 2003 Prospective semi-structured observational study to identify risk attributable to staff deployment, training and updating opportunities for midwives. British Medical Journal 327: 584

Chapter 5

Outcome of premature births
Alison Miller

The important thing to keep in sight is the vast majority of premature babies go on to lead happy healthy lives.[1]

INTRODUCTION

Prematurity is the major cause of neonatal deaths. According to the premature baby charity Bliss, babies born at 23 weeks have a 17% chance of survival, babies born at 24 weeks have a 39% chance of survival, whilst babies born at 25 weeks have a 50% chance of survival.[2] These figures do not take into account the morbidity of babies who survive.

Survival rates improve rapidly between 24 and 28 weeks, and by 28 weeks most babies are expected to survive. The Confidential Enquiries into Stillbirths and Deaths in Infancy (CESDI), therefore, selected a cohort of babies born alive at 27–28 weeks' gestation for their enquiry programme for 1998–2001.

Midwives play an important role in ensuring the appropriate care and management provided for women, which takes account of any increased risk factors. These factors can be identified at any stage during pregnancy and labour. This chapter is aimed at highlighting issues and recommendations from a midwifery perspective of the findings of the CESDI Project 27/28 Weeks report[3] specifically, but many of the recommendations can be applied to the care of mothers at risk of premature delivery.

AIMS OF THE ENQUIRY

There were two main aims of the project. First, to establish survival rates for babies born between 27^{+0} and 28^{+6} weeks' gestation. Second, to identify, through confidential enquiries, differences in standards of care that may contribute to the outcome for babies in this gestational category. In total, 3522 liveborn babies were notified and, of these, 88% were alive at day 28.

STUDY METHODOLOGY

As data regarding gestational age are not collected routinely within England, Wales or Northern Ireland, logbooks were provided for all labour wards and neonatal units within these areas. These were completed over a 2-year period: September 1998 to August 2000. Data were entered onto the labour ward logs of all babies born within the range 26^{+0}–29^{+6}. This was followed up by details of all babies at this gestation admitted to a neonatal unit being entered onto the neonatal logs (Table 5.1). The neonatal unit data recorded all admission, discharge and transfer details on babies up to 28 days post delivery. This provided a comprehensive picture of the different types of neonatal units in England, Wales and Northern Ireland, and high-lighted the inter-unit transfers of babies.

The 4-week gestational range of initial notification was used to maximize the appropriate inclusion of all babies. An algorithm was then applied to identify more accurately all babies within 27^{+0}–28^{+6} weeks, and these babies provided the final study denominator.

Confidential enquiries were also conducted on all babies in the study cohort who died within 28 days of birth and on a random selection of controls drawn from those who were surviving at 28 days.

Multidisciplinary panels carried out enquiry assessments at regional level. Panels comprised midwives, obstetricians, neonatal nurse specialists and neonatologists. Ideally, there were two members from each of these disciplines, but a minimum of one was accepted. Pathologists, community paediatricians, general practitioners (GPs) and observers (usually junior staff) were also invited to attend for educational purposes.

Table 5.1   Labour ward and neonatal unit data set recorded on notification

Topic	Details obtained
Ultrasound scan (USS)	Date of first USS <20 weeks' gestation
	Gestation at first USS <20 weeks (weeks and days)
Mother	Age
	Last menstrual period (LMP)
Delivery	Presentation
	Mode
Birth	Place of birth
	Clinical gestation at delivery (weeks and days)
	Date and time of delivery
Baby	Sex
	Number of babies in this pregnancy
	Birth order
	Birth weight (g)
	Life-threatening congenital malformation
Admission to neonatal unit	Name of previous unit or ward
	Date of admission to this unit
Paediatric assessment	Date at which the paediatrician assessed gestation
	Estimated gestation (weeks and days)
Transfer	Place and date of next transfer out of this unit or date of death

The important difference between the methodology used for this enquiry and previous CESDI enquiries was twofold: a case-control approach was used, and the obstetricians and midwives were blinded to the outcome and thus able to assess the standards of care based on the management given rather than outcome.

Analysis for this project was carried out using the case-control approach, which provided the opportunity for the analysis of this enquiry to include a comparison of the clinical factors in a group of babies who died with those in a group of babies who survived.

Enquiries were held on 366 deaths and a random sample of 395 babies who survived. Assessments were made against pre-defined national standards and guidelines set by professional bodies and also against good local practice criteria (Table 5.2).

Recommendations were developed by a recommendation advisory group (RAG) specifically convened for CESDI Project 27/28 Weeks, together with the use of the Delphi technique. The technique involves the recruitment of experts in a particular field and the repeated questioning of each group member, using sequential

Table 5.2 Specific topics addressed by the enquiry

Pre delivery
Administration of steroids
Management of chorioamnionitis
In-utero transfers
Fetal surveillance antenatally and in labour

Post delivery
Resuscitation
Early thermal care
Use of surfactants
Ventilatory and cardiovascular support
Management of infection
Transfers in the first 7 days of life

Pathology
Standard of post-mortem report
Personnel undertaking report
Contribution of post mortem to modification of clinical assessment
Neuropathological findings

General
Communication with parents
Communication between maternity and neonatal staff
Participation in trials
Record keeping
Deficiencies in organization

questionnaires. A statistical summary of group responses is prepared following each round of questions. This is used in developing the next round of questions, and is issued as feedback so that individuals may revise their views through awareness of overall responses, rather than through pressure from individuals. It has been suggested that group members, although they never meet, function as a nominal or focus group.[4]

FINDINGS OF CONFIDENTIAL ENQUIRIES INTO STILLBIRTHS AND DEATHS IN INFANCY PROJECT 27/28 WEEKS

Antenatal management

Maternal characteristics

The initial area of assessment sought to identify whether there were any maternal characteristics that could be identified antenatally that

Table 5.3   Demographic characteristics of mothers

	Mothers of babies who died (%)* n = 352	Mothers of babies who survived (%)* n = 371	Significance test p-value
Mean age in years [SD]	28.1 [6.2]	28.2 [6.5]	0.76 (ns)
Missing	1	2	
Ethnic origin			
White	251 (82.0)	256 (78.5)	0.32 (ns)
AfroCaribbean	18 (5.9)	29 (8.9)	
black African	11	15	
black Caribbean	7	12	
black other	0	2	
Asian	22 (7.2)	21 (6.4)	
Indian	8	8	
Pakistani	12	9	
Bangladeshi	2	4	
Chinese	4 (1.3)	5 (1.5)	
Other	11 (3.6)	15 (4.6)	
Missing	46	45	
Civil status			
Married	183 (55.3)	183 (51.1)	0.08 (ns)
Co-habiting	74 (22.4)	74 (20.7)	
Single	68 (20.5)	92 (25.7)	
Separated	1 (0.3)	4 (1.1)	
Divorced	5 (1.5)	5 (1.4)	
Missing	21	13	
Mother employed	181/303 (59.7)	208/331 (62.8)	0.47 (ns)
Father employed	221/262 (84.4)	248/285 (87.0)	0.44 (ns)

*The % is calculated from the number of mothers for which the information was available
ns, not significant

might predispose a mother to preterm labour (Table 5.3). This table shows some of the demographic data that were collected, and highlights any statistically significant differences. A p-value of less than 0.05 is thought to be significant.

Most of the maternal characteristics when related to outcome were similar for both groups of mothers. However, mothers of babies who died booked at a slightly earlier gestation, had early pre-labour rupture of membranes (PROM), and had an earlier occurrence of both preterm labour and bacteriuria. As routine early pregnancy information did not contain more detail about specific problems arising in pregnancy, it was difficult to identify those cases in which early specialist referral was appropriate.

There were three areas of notable difference in the characteristics of mothers associated with an increased risk of preterm birth at 27–28 weeks' gestation when compared to the maternity population of England, Wales and Northern Ireland: (1) the proportion of smokers, (2) the distribution of ethnicity and (3) multiple pregnancies.

One of the more interesting observations of the study found that 37% of mothers smoked some time during their pregnancy, in contrast to 19% of mothers in the Infant Feeding Survey 2000.[5] (The Infant Feeding Survey was based on a representative sample of all maternities in the UK during a comparable time period.) This large difference suggests a significantly increased risk of preterm birth and its associated complications to both mother and baby for women who smoke during pregnancy. Evidence shows that interventions from professionals are more effective in stopping people smoking than smokers using their own efforts to stop and that to give direct advice is better than doing nothing or giving self-help leaflets and contact information.[6] It is, therefore, important that adequate time is allocated at booking appointments for discussion of smoking habits in a non-judgmental way with the midwife, and the plan for support is offered throughout the pregnancy with the aid of the smoking cessation team, if available.

Advice regarding smoking and referral or guidance towards specialist services may be appropriate for both smokers and women from ethnic-minority groups. Whether community or hospital based, midwives are in the best position to build up a relationship of trust through which advice and direction to support services may be better accessed.

The study found that there were increased numbers of mothers from ethnic-minority groups (79% white) when compared with those in the Infant Feeding Survey 2000 (91% white),[5] suggesting ethnic origin may be important in the aetiology of preterm birth. This, however, did not reach statistical significance in the CESDI study. The importance of appropriate support where there are language barrier problems must be taken into account to ensure that all information regarding prompt identification of early labour and the mothers' self referral is provided and understood. Issues occurring within this group of women are highlighted in the midwifery-practice section of the Confidential Enquiries into Maternal Deaths (CEMD) report 1997–99.[7]

One in four maternities at 27/28 weeks' gestation was a multiple birth,[8] compared with 1 in 70 of all maternities.[9] Although in this CESDI project, survival proved to be equivalent for both singleton and multiple births (88%), there is evidence to suggest that babies from multiple pregnancies are much more likely to be born early and are over seven times more likely to die in the first month of life than a singleton baby.[10]

Assisted reproductive techniques have played a large part in the recent rapid increase in the proportion of multiple pregnancies.[9] The last report from the CEMD shows multiple pregnancies may be harmful to mothers as well as to babies. The report shows a mortality rate for mothers with twin pregnancy to be twice that of mothers of singletons and approximately 20 times greater for mothers with a triplet pregnancy.[7]

Recommendations

Midwives should be aware that structured interventions from them and nurses and also individual and group counselling are effective in helping women to stop smoking and should be included in their practice wherever possible.[6] Particular attention should be paid to those in higher risk groups.

Midwives caring for women with multiple pregnancies should be aware of the increased risks for both mothers and their babies and manage them proactively.

Place of delivery

The unit co-ordinators provided information at the start of the project about the types of maternity and neonatal units, grading them using standardized guidelines according to the level of care given within their unit.

It was interesting to find that there were no differences between the outcomes for babies of maternity or neonatal units graded using any of the following factors: place of delivery, type of maternity unit or neonatal facilities. This is in accordance with the previous national findings from the EPICure study[11] Project 27/28, which did not identify as part of its notification process the number of mothers transferred prior to delivery, but highlighted that 92% of the babies were born appropriately in hospitals providing neonatal intensive care. The assessments did identify that there is a general lack of adequate, clear national standards and guidelines for transfer for both mothers in premature labour and for babies following delivery.

Recommendations

- Any staff involved in the transfer process (in-utero or ex-utero) should be trained in transfer arrangements.
- A midwife should accompany any mother transferred in labour in a paramedic ambulance.

Babies' characteristics

Unlike the maternal characteristics, there were differences identified between the characteristics of the babies who survived compared to those of the babies who died. A higher risk of mortality was associated with being male, weighing less than the 5th centile and the presence of non-lethal congenital malformations noted within 28 days of birth. The Apgar scores and other measured characteristics showed significant differences between the babies who survived and those who died, suggesting that the group of babies that went on to die were more compromised at delivery. There are no specific recommendations reported from these findings. However, if these characteristics are identified at any stage in the antenatal period, midwives should put in place appropriate systems for correct referral and management of the mothers of these babies for their subsequent care.

The panel assessment of fetal well-being was extensive. It looked at the type of assessments made, adequacy of the assessment and then appropriateness of subsequent actions taken following various methods used. These included antenatal CTG, scan measurement, liquor volume, umbilical artery Dopplers and full biophysical profiles. In order to compare the differences between the two groups the crude odds ratio (OR) and the statistical significance (p-values) were calculated. In addition, an adjusted OR was calculated adjusting for babies who were below the 5th centile for weight (Table 5.4).

The enquiry findings showed a highly significant difference in deficiencies in fetal well-being assessment of babies who died (26%) compared with babies who survived (18%).

The findings relating to care provided by the midwife emphasized how essential it is that appropriate referrals are made and follow-up of care plans for subsequent management adhered to. Specifically, cardiotocographs (CTGs) were highlighted as being too brief to be adequately interpreted, of poor quality and the early gestation led to difficulties in accurate interpretation.

Because of the similarities in the characteristics of the mothers in both the cases and controls, it is difficult for clinicians to identify 'at-risk' babies during the antenatal period. However, identifying and appropriately managing the mother who is more likely to labour prematurely may reduce the risks of poor outcome for the baby.

Recommendations

All midwives should receive training and be aware of the indications for fetal well-being tests. Annual CTG training should include interpretation of the preterm CTG.

Table 5.4   Panel opinion: antepartum assessment of fetal well-being

	Babies who died (%)* $n = 366$	Babies who survived (%)* $n = 395$	Crude OR (95% CI) p-value	Adjusted OR** (95% CI) p-value
Inadequate assessment	91 (25.6)	69 (17.8)	1.59 (1.12–2.26) 0.01 sig	1.52 (1.03–2.24) 0.04 sig
Missing	11	8		
Inadequate interpretation	48 (14.1)	35 (9.3)	1.59 (1.00–2.53) 0.05 sig	1.42 (0.85–2.38) 0.18 ns
Missing	25	20		
Inappropriate action	86 (24.8)	55 (14.4)	1.95 (1.34–2.84) <0.001 sig	1.61 (1.08–2.42) 0.002 sig
Missing	19	14		
Deficiencies in seniority of staff	36 (11.5)	35 (10.3)	1.12 (0.69–1.84) 0.64 ns	0.92 (0.53–1.61) 0.77 ns
Missing	52	56		

*The % is calculated from the number of babies for which information was available
sig, significant; ns, not significant
**Adjusted for predelivery evidence of <5th centile

Every woman at this gestation should be seen by a consultant obstetrician within 24 hours of admission and have her plan of care reviewed. Midwives may need to ensure this referral is appropriately made.

Management of preterm labour

There were three aspects of the antenatal management of preterm labour that were assessed: prophylactic corticosteroids, chorioamnionitis and the use of tocolytics.

As previously stated, prematurity is one of the major causes of mortality and morbidity. The administration of steroids has been shown to reduce the risk of neonatal mortality and respiratory distress syndrome (RDS) by up to one-third.[11]

It was acknowledged that there was not always time to give corticosteroids and so the panel assessed the efforts made by health professionals to administer steroids. The findings showed that in this area management was suboptimal more frequently where the baby died (16%), than where the baby survived (11%). Although this difference only just failed to reach statistical significance, it suggests clinicians should be aware of these findings. The single most common reason for this assessment was failure by the health professionals to appreciate that corticosteroids were indicated. As there is always a midwife specifically allocated to the care of each woman, some of the responsibility for ensuring prompt prescription of steroids is made should lie with the midwife.

Evidence suggests that, although optimum benefit is gained when corticosteroids are given more than 24 hours but less than 7 days prior to delivery, it is likely that there is still some benefit when they are given outside that time limit, and, therefore, every effort should be made to administer steroids despite the possibility of imminent delivery.[12]

Although in this study clinical chorioamnionitis was not statistically associated with death or survival, other studies, together with a meta-analysis, have shown that cerebral palsy in premature infants may be associated with the presence of chorioamnionitis and maternal antibiotic.[13,14] Midwives should always ensure the first vaginal examination, required to confirm diagnosis of preterm labour and obtain microbiological specimens, is made using a speculum, as digital examination might theoretically increase the risk of ascending infection.

Although there is no clear evidence that the use of tocolytics improves pregnancy outcome, their use may be relevant in specific circumstances: to enable completion of a course of corticosteroids and to enable in-utero transfer of mother to a unit with appropriate neonatal facilities.[15]

Recommendations

- Midwives need to be aware both of the difficulties in diagnosis of preterm labour and the benefits of antenatal administration of steroids where women present with threatened preterm labour.

- Prompt referral to an obstetrician with appropriate expertise should be made in all cases of threatened preterm labour.

Intrapartum management

All deliveries occurring at 27–28 weeks' gestation are of high risk and demand rapid and effective co-ordination with the obstetric, neonatal and anaesthetic services. The latter is important, as the findings showed that the mode of most deliveries at this gestation was Caesarean section.

Nearly one-tenth of babies were delivered by upper-segment Caesarean section. It is essential that this incision is documented clearly, as this is likely to impact significantly on future pregnancies.[16]

Fluid balance was identified as an area of concern with regard to the risks associated with the combination of steroids, tocolytics and fluids. Midwives need to ensure that there is clarity and accuracy of documentation and record keeping regarding fluid balance throughout the care of the mother.

Recommendations

There is a need for high-risk delivery suite teams. These should include appropriately trained midwives. These teams should always take responsibility for the management of mothers in labour at 28 weeks' gestation or less.

The conduct of a vaginal delivery of a baby with a gestational age of 28 weeks or less should be performed or supervised by a senior member of the high-risk team.

Units should have in place local guidelines and standards concerning the management of intrapartum care of the mother and her preterm baby. These should be reviewed on a regular basis.

Immediate post-delivery resuscitation of the baby

Information was only available for 606 babies in the enquiry.

The enquiry identified a problem with the timely attendance of skilled staff at the delivery of preterm infants in 45% of deliveries. Issues around expertise in intubation were particularly highlighted and were more frequent in babies who died (14%) than in those babies who survived (9%). This may have been because babies who required intubation were more compromised.

Hypothermia on admission to the neonatal unit and deficiencies in the early thermal care were observed more frequently in babies who died.

The enquiry also highlighted poor documentation regarding the circumstances and personnel present at the time of delivery and during resuscitation. The guidelines on which the standard for assessment of personnel was based state that personnel present for resuscitation should include: an intermediate- or consultant-grade paediatrician, in addition to a junior paediatrician from the neonatal unit, and all should be present for the delivery.[17] However, it was particularly difficult to tell from the documentation which grades and what number of staff were in attendance at resuscitation, what their responsibilities were and at what stage of delivery they had arrived.

Recommendations

- The staff responsible for the immediate care of a baby born at 28 weeks' gestation or less should be trained in neonatal life support and at least one person present should be skilled in tracheal intubation.

- All labour ward and paediatric staff should be trained in the thermal care of infants during resuscitation, and the temperature in the delivery room should be at least 25°C.[18]

Neonatal management

As many midwives also practice in neonatal units, it is useful to complete the picture by giving an overview of the subsequent findings and recommendations, following assessment of the care of the premature baby after delivery and up to 7 days of life.

There were five main areas of focus following delivery of these premature babies: early thermal care, surfactant therapy, ventilatory support, cardiovascular support and management of infection.

Hypothermia has been shown to be a cause of both increased mortality and morbidity in the premature baby as they are at particular risk due to evaporation heat loss from their skin.[19] The standard for this assessment was that the baby's temperature should be above 36°C on admission to the neonatal unit.[20] This standard is based on accepted good practice and the project organizers noted that there is little evidence-based guidance regarding management of early thermal care of the neonate. It was appreciated by the panel members that following intensive resuscitation, handling and transfer, this was a very high standard to meet, together with the increased likelihood that these interventions are more likely to affect the more critically ill babies. However, after removing data on babies who died in the first 24 hours, the babies who subsequently died had a mean temperature significantly lower than the babies who survived (59% v 73%, $p < 0.001$), showing an association between hypothermia and death. Seen as an isolated factor it is even more important to appreciate the importance of proactive management in keeping the baby warm.

Recommendations

- All labour ward and paediatric staff should be trained in the thermal care of infants at resuscitation.
- All transfers of preterm infants should take place in a warmed transport incubator.

- Temperature should be recorded and documented within 30 minutes of delivery and then at least 4 hourly.
- Continuous temperature recording is necessary for all infants requiring intensive care.
- Incubators should be capable of maintaining appropriate temperature and humidity and should be checked regularly.

Surfactant therapy

Premature babies have immature lungs that are deficient in surfactant and can lead to increased mortality and morbidity due to RDS. Surfactant administered via the trachea can reduce this risk by 40% and should be administered as soon after birth as is practical to all intubated babies.[21–23] This evidence has led to national guidelines that ensure that surfactant administration is routine in the care of the preterm baby, and possibly reflects the high assessment of this standard – 96% of intubated babies received surfactant. However, only 61% of cases were deemed to have received surfactant as soon as was practicable. This may be due to surfactant being administered only to babies considered to be at risk of RDS rather than being administered prophylactically, although the criteria for 'at risk' are uncertain.

Deficiencies in the administration of surfactant therapy were identified in 32% of babies who died compared with 21% of the babies who survived and this difference was statistically significant (Fig. 5.1 & Table 5.5). Most babies who survived did not receive

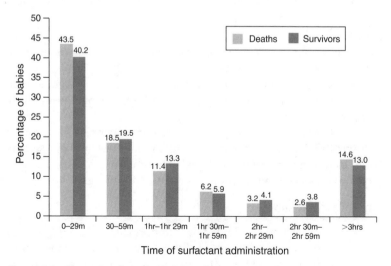

Figure 5.1   Time of surfactant administration

Table 5.5   Reasons why surfactant was not administered

Reason	Babies who died ($n = 41$)	Babies who survived ($n = 46$)
Baby died or too unwell	19	0
Not at risk of RDS	4	35
Miscellaneous	1	2
Should have been given according to standards	2	0
Cannot tell	3	4
No reason provided by panel	12	5

surfactant because they were not thought to be at risk of RDS, were being nursed in air or required minimal ventilation.

The overall findings for the assessments of these standards suggest that if all babies were given surfactant within 1 hour of birth, there is likelihood that survival rates could be improved.

Recommendations

- All units should implement the national guidance on the timing and gestation at which prophylactic surfactant should be administered and the indications for repeat doses.

- Units should ensure that there are explicit guidelines readily available regarding the administration of surfactants.

- Documentation of surfactant therapy should be clear and explicit.

Ventilatory support

Most babies born at 27–28 weeks' gestation will need some form of ventilatory support due to the increased risk of RDS. The panels were asked to assess a variety of different aspects of care that together aim to achieve adequate gas exchange without impairment to pulmonary or cerebral functions.

There were 83% of babies who required ventilatory support following delivery. The main concerns highlighted by the assessors were: lack of management plan, delays or failures in responding to blood gas results and inappropriate ventilator settings.

Cardiovascular support

The aim of providing cardiovascular support is to reduce the risks of peri/intraventricular haemorrhage, ischaemic cerebral lesions, poor long-term neuro-developmental outcomes and mortality in the preterm.[24] To do this the baby should have regular blood-pressure measurements and any events of hypotension should be treated immediately if there is evidence of poor perfusion.[23]

The study found that the mismanagement of cardiovascular support was twice as likely not to meet the standards in babies who died compared with babies who lived to 28 days. This difference was maintained when the data were adjusted for severity of illness of the baby at 5 minutes following birth.

Management of infection

Babies below 28 weeks' gestation are inevitably at increased risk of infection, due to immaturity of the immune system. They are also more likely to be exposed to maternal infection causing the onset of preterm labour and have much more likelihood of being subject to invasive treatments following birth.[25] Again, the sick baby is much more at risk.

The panels found the standards for management of infection were generally high and were not associated with outcome. The most notable area where deficiencies were identified was delay in administration of antibiotics.

Communication and record keeping

As with all CESDI enquiries, assessments considered the communication and documentation standards throughout the care of each woman and, unfortunately, again many comments were made regarding deficiencies in these areas. The most notable for midwives were both the frequency with which mothers were apparently not seen by a member of the neonatal team prior to delivery, even when there was a clear time between diagnosis of preterm labour and delivery, and poor communication with the mother before the birth regarding the planned current and future management to be given. Attention must again be drawn to the findings of the CESDI 8th annual report regarding the need for clearly documented plans for care and the ongoing need to follow and update those plans appropriately. This reiterates the benefits of having one set of multidisciplinary notes, which enable plans to be actioned with continuity and consistency by all carers.[26]

Recommendations

- Formal communication should occur at least daily between the obstetric, midwifery and neonatal staff.

- All women should have a lead midwife who takes responsibility for updating the rest of the team and maintaining effective communication with the mother of the baby.

- Departments and trusts should ensure that their record design conforms to the good features of good record design as specified by the Nursing and Midwifery Council.[26]

SUMMARY

Outcomes for babies at 27–28 weeks' gestation have been identified as better than was initially expected. However, there was no scope within this enquiry to investigate the morbidity of the babies who survived and, therefore, the survival rates must be interpreted with caution.

With the increased survival opportunities for these babies, midwives and neonatal nurses play an important role in increasing the chances of good outcome following live delivery – both with regard to mortality and morbidity. Although this project looks solely at mortality, many of the recommendations made, if acted upon, have the possibility of reducing both the mortality and morbidity rates for this group of babies.

The aim of this enquiry was to identify areas of suboptimal care; however, it must also be noted that many of the assessments and comments made by the panelists were positive and praised the standards of care these women received.

References

1. Wood NS, Marlow N, Costeloe K et al. 2000 Neurologic and developmental disability after extremely preterm birth. EPICure Study Group. New England Journal of Medicine 343: 378–384
2. http://www.bliss.org.uk/about/facts.asp
3. CESDI 2003 Project 27/28 An enquiry into quality and care and its effect on the survival of babies born at 27–28 weeks. The Stationery Office, London
4. Beech B 1999 Go the extra mile – use the Delphi technique. Journal of Nursing Management 7: 281–288
5. IFS 2002 Infant feeding survey 2000 The Stationery Office, London
6. Lancaster T, Stead L, Silagy C, Sowden A 2000 Effectiveness of intervention to help people stop smoking. Findings from the Cochrane Library. British Medical Journal 321: 355–358
7. Lewis G, Drife J (eds) 2001 Why mothers die 1997–1999, 5th report of the confidential enquiry into maternal deaths in the United Kingdom. Royal College of Obstetricians and Gynaecologists Press, London
8. Maternal and Child Health Research Consortium 2001 CESDI 8th annual report. Department of Health, London
9. Chapple J 2001 Perinatal mortality. In: Chamberlain G, Steer P (eds). Turnbull's Obstetrics 3rd edn. Churchill Livingstone, Edinburgh, pp. 729–741

10. Macfarlane A, Mugford M 2000 Birth counts: statistics of pregnancy and childbirth. The Stationery Office, London, p. 181

11. Costeloe K, Hennessy E, Gibson A, Marlow N, Wilikinson AR 2000 The EPICure study: outcomes to discharge from hospital for infants born at the threshold of viability. Pediatrics 106: 659–671

12. Crowley P 2002 Prophylactic corticosteroids for preterm birth. Cochrane Library, Issue 1. Update Software, Oxford

13. O'Shea TM, Klinepeter KL, Dillard RG 1998 Prenatal events and the risk of cerebral palsy in the very low birth weight infants. American Journal of Epidemiology 147: 632–369

14. Wu YW, Colford Jr JM 2000 Chorioamnionitis as a risk factor for cerebral palsy: a meta-analysis. Journal of the American Medical Association 284: 2996–2997

15. Royal College of Obstetricians and Gynaecologists 1997 Beta-agonists for the care of women in preterm labour. Guideline no. 7. Royal College of Obstetricians and Gynaecologists, London

16. Halperin ME, Moore DC, Hannah WJ 1988 Classical versus low-segment transverse incision for preterm caesarean section: maternal complications and outcome of subsequent pregnancies. British Journal of Obstetrics and Gynaecology 95: 990–996

17. British Paediatric Association 1993 Neonatal resuscitation. British Paediatric Association, London

18. World Health Organization 1997 Thermal protection of the newborn, WHO/RHT/MSM/97.2. World Health Organization, Geneva

19. Bruck K 1992 Neonatal thermoregulation. In: Polin R, Fox WW (eds). Fetal and neonatal physiology. WB Saunders, Philadelphia, pp. 448–515

20. Joint Working Group of the British Association of Perinatal Medicine and Research Unit of the Royal College of Paediatrics and Child Health 1992 Development of audit measures and guidelines for good practice in the management of neonatal respiratory distress syndrome. Archives of Disease in Childhood 67: 1221–1227

21. Soll RF, Morley CJ 1998 Prophylactic surfactant vs. treatment with surfactant (Cochrane Review). Cochrane Library, Issue 2. Update Software, Oxford

22. Soll RF, Morley CJ 2001 Prophylactic versus selective use of surfactant for preventing morbidity and mortality in preterm infants (Cochrane Review). Cochrane Library, Issue 1. Update Software, Oxford

23. British Association of Perinatal Medicine 1999 Guidelines for the management of respiratory distress syndrome. British Association of Perinatal Medicine, London

24. Osborn DA, Evans N 2001 Early volume expansion for the prevention of morbidity and mortality in the very preterm infants (Cochrane Review). Cochrane Library, Issue 2. Update Software, Oxford

25. Hall M, Ironton R 1999 Infection. In: Levvitt G, Harvey D, Cooke R (eds). Practical perinatal care: the baby under 1000 g. Butterworth Heinemann, Oxford

26. Nursing and Midwifery Council 2002 Guidelines for records and record-keeping. Nursing and Midwifery Council, London

Chapter 6

Rare adverse events

Melanie J. Gompels and Grace Edwards

A principle feature of the enquiries is the ability to highlight aspects of care that traditional scientific studies have difficulty in eliciting.[1]

INTRODUCTION

There are a number of deaths that occur due to rare obstetric events. One of the benefits of collecting information at national level is that these events can be pooled to determine if there are general lessons that can be learnt. Confidential Enquiries into Stillbirths and Deaths in Infancy (CESDI) enabled data to be collated on a national scale, which, in turn, led to the identification of relatively rare clusters of adverse outcomes. Broader lessons may be learned about the management of rare events that an individual midwife may not have experienced or a single case may not highlight. As discussed in Chapter 4, the CESDI 4th annual report found that, of the one in ten normally formed deaths in 1994 and 1995 weighing over 1 kg, over two-thirds were potentially avoidable if a different course of action had been taken.[2]

Over 1000 cases were enquired nationally, and from these three particular areas were reviewed in the focus groups contained in the CESDI 5th annual report: planned home birth, ruptured uterus and shoulder dystocia.[1] Breech birth is also considered a relatively rare event that may result in an adverse outcome for the fetus. The incidence of breech presentation is approximately 3–4% of all births, and has long been associated with poor outcomes, and so these deaths are also considered in this chapter. Although such deaths make up less than 10% of those reported to CESDI, these rare adverse events are considered largely avoidable.

Unfortunately, due to the lack of national denominator data on all births, trend analysis of national survival rates associated with adverse outcomes, which involves a comparison of the prevalence of risk factors or management strategies for these rare events, is precluded.

Nationally specialist multidisciplinary focus groups were formed comprising obstetricians, midwives, general practitioners (GPs), paediatricians, one public health specialist and one lay representative. The cases were independently reviewed by two members of each group, specialist interests were balanced, and questionnaires were completed.

The panel graded the severity of the suboptimal care using the criteria adopted for the regional confidential enquiries, which are:

* 0 – No suboptimal care
* I – Suboptimal care, but different management would have made no difference
* II – Suboptimal care, different management MIGHT have made a difference
* III – Different management WOULD REASONABLY BE EXPECTED to have made a difference.

The purpose of each group was to try to reduce the number of avoidable adverse outcomes by highlighting areas of concern and making recommendations for best practice for local maternity units and healthcare professionals based on a combination of published evidence and consensus within the groups.

This chapter focuses on the midwifery aspects of the report findings on each type of adverse event. Specific points of suboptimal care, implications and recommendations for midwifery practice and management are highlighted.

Midwives need to recognize that potential adverse events may occur in any woman for whom they care, and they need to have the expertise to act appropriately. Additionally, midwives must be able to provide advice to women to enable them to make informed decisions, and must support them in their choice.

PLACE OF DELIVERY

There is a wide variation in the home-birth rate throughout the UK, ranging from 1% to over 20%.[3] This is mainly due to the widespread professional and public belief that birth in hospital is safer than home birth, but there is no evidence to support this belief in women with straightforward pregnancies.

Planned home birth has been shown to have good outcomes for both mothers and babies. A major study of almost 6000 women who planned home births found that they had around 50% less Caesarean sections, instrumental delivery and significantly fewer post-partum haemorrhages than a comparative group of women planning hospital birth.[4] There are also a number of research papers that highlight the practical and emotional benefits of home birth,[5] and there is evidence to show that women who have a planned home birth have less interventions such as Caesarean section, forceps or ventouse delivery.[6]

Despite this, by the end of the 20th century, less than 2% of deliveries in England, Wales and Northern Ireland were born at home.[7] Home birth had become unusual as a planned place of delivery due to the centralization of maternity services. Consequently, a decreasing number of midwives have sufficient experience in assisting women to give birth at home.

Within the CESDI, planned home-birth deaths, when compared with the 'overall' care grades of enquiries held on the 1994/5 cases, were found to be no more at risk of suboptimal care than other deaths ($p = 0.37$). Although it would be considered unethical and impractical to carry out a randomized controlled trial into home versus hospital births,[8] a recent meta-analysis on the safety of home birth concluded that planned home birth should be offered to all low-risk women.[9] However, there are still lessons that can be learnt from the findings of this review of planned home births.

The 5th CESDI report identified 22 deaths at home or substantially home-supervised labours for further retrospective casenote review. Half of the deaths ($n = 11$) were stillborn and the remainder of the deaths ($n = 11$) were classified as neonatal deaths. Of the 11 stillbirths, three were born at home, one in transit to hospital, and seven in hospital. Eight neonatal deaths were born at home and three neonatal deaths in hospital following transfer.

The CESDI review highlighted that some women experienced difficulty in obtaining professional support for home delivery, or that there was delay in calling for support when labour had commenced. Table 6.1 shows each case categorized into one of four levels of obstetric risk to enable low-risk women to be identified and to highlight the

Table 6.1 Category of obstetric risk in relation to stillbirths and neonatal deaths

	Category	Stillbirth	Neonatal death
A	Low obstetric risk criteria for home birth were not breached. Midwifery and medical professionals were fully supportive of the chosen place of delivery.	7	4
B	Low obstetric risk criteria for home birth were breached. The professions concerned recognized the breach, but at least one midwife or doctor willingly agreed to support home birth.	2	4
C	Low obstetric risk criteria for home birth were not breached, however, there was no formal professional agreement to support a home birth. Professions made plans for home birth support in order to comply with a duty of care.	2	2
D	Low obstetric risk criteria for home birth were breached and there was no formal professional agreement of support. Plans were made for home birth support in order to comply with a duty of care.	0	1

frequency of death. In one-third of cases, midwives were required to support women who had chosen to deliver at home despite not fulfilling the low obstetric risk criteria.

The enquiries highlighted a number of communication issues with home deliveries: in three cases, women in labour had difficulties in contacting their named midwives; in one instance, a 'back-up' hospital midwife was delayed due to unfamiliarity with the area; and in other cases, the appropriate individuals on the labour ward at the receiving hospital were not informed.

The deaths associated with home birth demonstrated that midwives often did not anticipate problems. In a number of cases, there was difficulty in confirming the presence of a fetal heart rate. There was also mention of considerable delay in seeking help or arranging transfer. There were also mentions in the records of fetal bradycardia and/or the passage of meconium with no subsequent action. Inadequate neonatal resuscitation was mentioned as a contributory factor in four of the 22 cases. The lack of availability of basic resuscitation equipment, such as bag and mask suggests inadequate preparation for this potential hazard. Additionally, an emergency situation was often compounded by undue delay in ambulance response times or long transfer times to the maternity unit. There were also issues around poor record keeping. In several of the cases there was a lack of adequate recording of the fetal heart rate, maternal vital signs (temperature, pulse, blood pressure) and progress of labour.

Overall, the enquiry process for these cases identified suboptimal care in 77% of the home births. This is comparable to the 69% in all intrapartum-related deaths reviewed in the 1994/5 confidential enquiries.[1]

Recommendations

Although the number of deaths is small, it is still possible to make recommendations for midwifery practice.

Informed choice

Local, evidenced-based guidelines should be developed around planned home births by all staff, and should include user group representatives.

Communication

A fixed-line telephone or mobile phone should be available. The woman should have clear instructions of who to contact if her named midwife is not available. Hospital staff and ambulance staff should be notified of planned home births in their area.

Detection of problems

The use of a partogram is the simplest method of ensuring that comprehensive records of vital signs and progress in labour are completed.

Transfer arrangements

Arrangements for transfer to hospital should be made at the earliest indication by the professional present at the time. Following transfer directly to labour ward, the most experienced staff should be forewarned of the transfer and be available for immediate assessment, including paediatric and anaesthetic staff available on site to enable an immediate operative delivery, if indicated.

Resuscitation

All midwives attending home births should have appropriate equipment for neonatal resuscitation and have regular updates and practical sessions in its use. Midwives have a professional duty of care to attend women, and support their choice of place of birth even when this conflicts with midwifery advice. The supervisor of midwives should ensure that the agreed local policies are easily available to all practising midwives within their supervisory jurisdiction. The local policy should provide support for the midwife and ensure that appropriate experience, training and support is available.

RUPTURED UTERUS

Uterine rupture is thought to occur in as many as one in 140 women who labour with a pre-existing uterine scar.[10] Forty-two infant deaths associated with uterine rupture were reviewed by assessors and summarized in the CESDI 5th annual report.[1]

Uterine rupture accounted for significantly more suboptimal care grade 3 deaths than other deaths. The panels considered that uterine rupture resulting in the death of the baby as an avoidable event in most cases.

Maternal haemorrhage is one of the major causes of maternal death.[11] Although none occurred in this group of uterine ruptures, nine women required a hysterectomy, and four cases presented following delivery due to maternal collapse.

Midwives need to be alert to antenatal risk factors known to predispose women to uterine rupture. The prevalence of obesity (BMI > 30) has increased in the UK over the past 10 years. In 1995 only 14% of the female population aged 16–54 years were considered obese,[12] compared with 20% of women in 1999.[13] However, obesity existed in nearly half (46%) of the cases of uterine rupture. Previous Caesarean section accounted for 70% of ruptured uterus, and within this group nearly two-thirds were induced – mainly by prostaglandins.

The national induction rate for all labours is over 20%[14] and is probably lower in women with a pre-existing scar. However, within the ruptured uterus group, induction occurred in 60% (18/30), which indicates that it may be a notable risk factor in this group.

The dose regimes followed for prostaglandin use were, in general, within the recommended range.[15, 16] Prostaglandin was the sole agent in 14 of the 18 inductions involving a pre-existing scar. The prostaglandin dosage was repeated in 10 of the 17 cases. Multiparous women were induced by prostaglandin solely in five cases, of these, two women received doses (2 mg) above the initial recommended dose of 1 mg. Syntocinon was used in one-quarter of the cases to augment labour due to diminished contractions and slow progress at or near full dilatation.

During labour and delivery midwives need to be vigilant regarding the presence of multiple warning signs such as scar pain, vaginal bleeding, poor progress (<1 cm/hr) or fetal distress lasting more than 1 hour. In addition, there may be other clinical signs, such as maternal tachycardia or shock. However, in half of the cases, uterine rupture occurred at or near full dilatation, and in five women the second stage of labour lasted more than 2 hours.

Midwives must consider preterm uterine rupture as a possible cause requiring admission for preterm labour. Although preterm uterine rupture is rare, within the 42 cases reviewed, three baby deaths involved women who had previous Caesarean sections, and required admission for possible preterm labour.

Four main themes of concern are identifiable from over 100 comments made by the assessors:

1. Antenatal management concerns regarding communication of delivery plans and the involvement of senior staff.

2. Inappropriate inductions, use of both prostaglandin and syntocinon.

3. A lack of adequate assessment of fetal well-being, maternal surveillance and recognition of uterine rupture.

4. Organizational failures including a lack of supervision of staff, inappropriate trials of scar in non-labour ward environments, and delay in arranging transfer to operating theatres.

Ruptured uterus is an avoidable adverse event which, with awareness and experience, midwives may be able to deal with in a more anticipatory manner. Although consultants were frequently criticized, the need for senior experienced involvement by midwives at key stages is stressed.

Recommendations

If a woman has a uterine scar, the care plan should include:

- a plan for delivery and induction involving a documented discussion with an experienced obstetrician
- attentive intrapartum fetal and maternal surveillance in a setting where the baby can be delivered within 30 minutes
- no more than one dose of prostaglandin, unless great vigilance is exercised
- local guidelines regarding the augmentation of labour
- local guidelines regarding the setting and standards of intrapartum fetal and maternal surveillance in women with a uterine scar.

Training issues

All involved in the intrapartum care of women must be aware of the factors that may lead to uterine rupture. In particular, they must recognize that women with a uterine scar are 'high risk' and should be managed appropriately.

All involved in the intrapartum care of women should undergo training in the use and interpretation of CTGs.

SHOULDER DYSTOCIA

Although there are various definitions of shoulder dystocia, 'true' shoulder dystocia is rare. As the CESDI database only collates information on deaths, all deaths in which there was evidence of shoulder dystocia were reviewed. The CESDI 5th annual report identified 56 cases where shoulder dystocia was perceived as delaying delivery.

Most cases of shoulder dystocia are unexpected, consequently, the midwife is usually the lead healthcare professional available to identify the problem and summon emergency assistance to expedite delivery. Delay in delivery of the body increases the risk of fetal demise within a relatively short space of time (less than 5 minutes). In 65% of cases the midwife was the lead professional at delivery. The use of a combination of traction and McRoberts' manoeuvre was successful in delivery of the shoulders in 75% of cases.

In the 56 cases reviewed, two-thirds were deemed avoidable, i.e. the enquiry panel felt that there were avoidable factors that would have been amenable to different management that would have altered the outcome ($p < 0.001$).

Professional opinion suggests the prediction of shoulder dystocia during the antenatal period is possible by adopting a risk assessment approach. In practice, the review of cases found that the predictive value of classical risk factors was low. Severe obesity (BMI > 40) was present in 11% (six cases), impaired glucose tolerance was present in 8% (four cases), and a prediction of a large baby was made in 40% ($n = 22$). Midwives need to recognize that shoulder dystocia often occurs where there are no apparent risk factors, and that a high level of anticipation and use of intuition may be the best approach in planning care.[17]

Recognition of fetal distress during labour and delivery was a recurring theme of the CESDI 4th annual report. Within the shoulder dystocia focus group, fetal distress was only recognized in 26% ($n = 14$) of cases prior to delivery of the head. The reason why

47% (21) of stillborn babies failed to respond to resuscitation after a 5 minutes or less interval between delivery of the body and the head, can probably be explained by the preceding unrecognized hypoxic stress that renders a fetus less tolerant of further hypoxia due to shoulder dystocia. Underestimates in the head–body delivery interval may also help to explain the rapidity of fetal demise, as 70% of babies showed no signs of life at birth. The CESDI 4th annual report highlighted that the quality of maternity records needs to be improved; clear documentation of risk factors and management plans is needed to enable accurate record keeping by midwives and healthcare professionals.

Avoiding delay in expediting delivery following recognition of shoulder dystocia is paramount. Maternity units need to have in place clear action plans or 'fire drills' for the management of shoulder dystocia that are regularly practiced in a multiprofessional environment.[17]

Perinatal autopsy assists healthcare professionals in understanding the causes of fetal demise, helps with the identification of undetected abnormalities, and, most importantly, may allay parental concerns regarding the circumstances of death. The Royal Colleges of Pathology and Obstetrics and Gynaecology recommend that 75% of fetal and infant deaths should undergo an autopsy.[18] Within the shoulder dystocia group, there was a disappointingly low rate (45%) and poor quality (32%) of autopsy. Regional studies indicate that, increasingly, parents refuse consent in up to one-third of deaths, and healthcare professionals feel unable to request a post mortem in 20% of cases.[19] Midwives need to ensure that they have a clear understanding of the value of post mortem and should be trained in approaching parents in a sympathetic manner towards reaching an informed decision.

Recommendations

- Since shoulder dystocia is a rare emergency, a high level of awareness and training of all birth attendants is necessary.
- The 'fire drill' should include clear instructions for calling the appropriate professional.
- The accepted sequence of clinical manoeuvres should be clearly presented in local guidelines.

BREECH BIRTH

Breech presentation at term occurs in approximately 3–4% of all births, and has long been associated with poor outcomes. Breech birth is also considered a relatively rare event that may result in a adverse outcome for the baby. In a recent international multicentred randomized controlled trial, there was over a 3% risk of an adverse perinatal outcome associated with planned breech vaginal delivery compared with a planned Caesarean.[20] However, some critics of the trial suggest that breech vaginal delivery outcomes are no worse in low perinatal mortality countries where accurate pre-labour assessment identifies small-for-gestational-age fetuses.[21]

The manual manipulation of a breech presentation by external cephalic version (ECV) has been found to reduce breech births by over 50%[22] and is recommended in uncomplicated term breech pregnancies.[23] In practice, the technique is not universally offered by healthcare professionals, or taken up by the woman. ECV is perceived, by both practitioner and future parents, as carrying additional risks such as cord prolapse, cord entanglement that may result in placental abruption, and feto-maternal haemorrhage, but these are unproven.

Table 6.2   HELPER mnemonic

A. Help
1. Call for Help
B. Episiotomy
1. Cut a generous episiotomy
C. Legs
1. Position with McRoberts' manoeuvre for 30–60 seconds
D. Pressure applied over bladder (suprapubic)
1. Oblique downward and anterior pressure for 30–60 seconds
E. Enter
1. Position hands in position
a. two fingers by anterior shoulder
b. two fingers by posterior shoulder
2. Rubin manoeuvre: rotate counter-clockwise for 30–60 seconds
3. Wood-Screw manoeuvre: rotate clockwise for 30–60 seconds
F. Remove the posterior arm
1. Roll the patients to hands and knees
2. Repeat the above procedure
Avoid
A. Fundal pressure
B. Excessive traction
C. Twisting or bending neck

Errata

Within *Adverse Outcomes in Maternity Care* there is a reference to the HELPERR mnemonic devised by the Advanced Life Support in Obstetrics (ALSO)(page 106). The reference is meant to inform the reader of the benefits of using mnemonics in emergency care, but also to direct readers to further reading. A more comprehensive table suggested by ALSO is shown on our website www.elsevierhealth.com

The paragraph on page 107 should read:

The use of the 'HELPERR' mnemonic (Table 6.2) may be a good method in ensuring a co-ordinated multi-disciplinary response to shoulder dystocia.

and should have been placed on page 105.

As many breech deliveries are unrecognized, present late, occur with the second twin, or are preterm, midwives need to have acquired the skills in recognition and delivery of breech presentation. The use of the 'HELPER'[24] mnemonic (Table 6.2) may be a good method in ensuring a co-ordinated multi-disciplinary response to vaginal breech deliveries.

More importantly, some women may choose a vaginal delivery in preference to a Caesarean delivery and need to be supported in their decision by midwives.

SUBOPTIMAL CARE

Three overall themes of sub-optimal care are identifiable from the adverse outcome enquiries: adequate risk assessment, communication and record keeping.

Of the three groups, ruptured uterus was identified as having the greater proportion of substandard care that was considered avoidable. Both ruptured uterus- and shoulder dystocia-related deaths had a significantly greater proportion of grade 3 suboptimal factors when compared with other deaths enquired in 1994/5 ($p < 0.001$).

Care during labour and delivery were the most commonly cited concerns in over 70% of cases. A sequence of a lack of recognition and action to problems were compounded by communication lapses in 25% of deaths. Midwives were found to be responsible for 22% of suboptimal care comments in 46% of cases compared with obstetricians, 36% of comments affecting 60% of cases. The proportions most likely reflected the relative involvement of each professional group in provision of intrapartum care, although any one case often had failures by more that one professional group.

In the ruptured uterus group, eight cases were considered to have substandard casenotes, and were retrospectively completed in two instances. The safe storage of cardiotocographs and partograms was lacking in 23 cases. Misinterpretation of progress in labour may be due to discrepancies in timings due to variation in practitioner familiarity and use of the partogram. For example, fetal cephalic decent within the pelvis (fifths palpable) and the level identified above or below the ischial spines are not highlighted on many partograms.

Overall, these adverse outcomes were found to have more frequent and serious factors of substandard care.

Table 6.3 details a summary of the care grades allocated to all cases in the CESDI 4th annual report by the panels initially, and the subsequent grade when reviewed by the focus groups in detail.

Table 6.3 Summary of grades of suboptimal care for all enquiries, intrapartum-related deaths, planned home birth, ruptured uterus and shoulder dystocia

	All enquiries 1994–1995		Intrapartum deaths		Planned home birth		Ruptured uterus		Shoulder dystocia	
Total cases (n)	1266	100%	873	100%	22	100%	42	100%	56	100%
Ungraded	8	0.5%	4	0.5%	0		0		0	
Grade 0 or 1	392	31%	195	22%	5	23%	2	6%	6	11%
Grade 2	326	26%	219	25%	7	32%	8	19%	13	23%
Grade 3	540	43%	455	52%	10	45%	32	75%	37	66%

Grade 0 = No suboptimal care
Grade 1 = Suboptimal care, but different management would have made NO difference to the outcome
Grade 2 = Suboptimal care that MIGHT have made a difference to the outcome
Grade 3 = Suboptimal care where a different course of action WOULD REASONABLY BE EXPECTED to have made a difference to the outcome

Recommendations: key messages

Adverse outcomes in maternity care remain relatively rare events, but are considered largely avoidable in the majority of cases. The CESDI 5th annual report brought together three areas that midwives may encounter that potentially may result in a death: homebirth, ruptured uterus and shoulder dystocia. Vaginal breech birth is also considered in this chapter, as it has traditionally been associated with poor outcomes.

The key messages from the recommendations from adverse events in maternity care, as they relate to the organizational provision of midwifery care, the individual midwife practitioner, and meeting the needs of woman are summarized below. The full CESDI 5th annual report details these further, and can be obtained from the CEMACH website: *www.cemach.org.uk*

Provision of care: organizational

Protocols and guidelines

Midwives, working in any setting, need to work with professional colleagues to develop local evidence-based protocols and guidelines, e.g. defining high-obstetric-risk criteria and level of subsequent management, location of delivery, and augmentation of labour.

Increasingly, national guidelines and effective evidence-based research needs to be actively incorporated into everyday midwifery practice, e.g. National Institute for Clinical Excellence (NICE) guidelines on fetal monitoring and induction of labour.

Embracing clinical governance agenda by promoting a culture of reporting and patient safety

Each unit should also have an internal system of reviewing adverse events in a multidisciplinary environment, regardless of the outcome, to learn important practice points.

Surveillance, monitoring and risk recognition

Within maternity organizations, midwives need to review their efforts at identifying potential risk of an adverse outcome. A culture needs to be created by midwives whereby care is appropriately targeted to potential high-risk women. Ongoing midwifery care needs to be regularly reviewed as the woman progresses through her pregnancy, to ensure that delays are minimized, and referrals are timely. For example, the use of the partogram to record maternal and fetal progress in labour, and fetal Doppler should be available to midwives to ensure they are able to detect suspected fetal distress.

'Fire drills' and mnemonics

The use of 'fire drills' and mnemonics may be a good method in ensuring a coordinated multidisciplinary response to rare adverse events. These need to be regularly practiced in a multiprofessional environment.

Supervision

The role of senior midwives to be available to support newly qualified or junior staff needs to be transparent, clearly defined and reviewed regularly.

Communication

There should be clearly documented guidelines for summoning assistance of the multidisciplinary team.

Personal professional accountability and practice

These may be categorized as individual practitioner responsibilities and professional training issues.

Training

Support should be available to encourage reflection and development of practice, e.g. regular training in the appropriate use of cardiotocographs should be mandatory for all staff.

Equipment and its use

Neonatal resuscitation equipment and training should be available to all midwives planning to undertake a home delivery. Midwives need to ensure they undertake regular updates in the use of the bag and mask in resuscitation.

Maintaining skills and competence levels

There should be alerts to risk factors, which can be multiple but are not always predictive, e.g. obesity, multiparity, induction of labour. Although uterine rupture is rare, midwives need to be able to readily identify the risk factors of uterine rupture, especially when caring for the increasing number of women with a previous scar.

Record keeping

These should be clear and contemporaneous. The importance of maintaining contemporaneous records has been cited in earlier CESDI reports. Maternity units are also responsible for their safe storage. Despite these recommendations, record keeping remains a reoccurring theme that leaves healthcare professionals vulnerable to medical negligence claims. Midwives need to familiarize themselves with the new guidelines for records and record keeping issued by the Nursing and Midwifery Council (NMC).[25]

Post mortem

Perinatal autopsy assists parents and healthcare professionals in understanding the causes of fetal demise, as well as the identification of undetected abnormalities. Midwives need to ensure that they have a clear understanding of the value of post mortem and should be trained in assisting parents making an informed decision.

Meeting the needs of women

There are four key areas identified:

1. Communication: delivery plans and obtaining professional support.
2. Active advocacy role within organization.

3. Services should meet women's needs.
4. Continuity of care.

Midwives need to advise and assist women to make an informed choice in deciding the place of delivery which should be evidence based. If a home birth is planned, the midwife needs to ensure that the mother has complete confidence in the midwife's support, so she does not delay in notifying when labour has commenced.

Midwives attending women planning to deliver at home need a mobile telephone; additionally, wherever possible, women planning to deliver at home should also have a telephone available. The named midwife responsible for the arrangements of the home births must ensure the woman is aware of the back-up arrangements and who to contact in the event she is not immediately available. Midwives should undertake a 'dry-run' in the case of unusual or isolated addresses, and inform ambulance services of planned home births in their area.

References

1. Maternal and Child Health Research Consortium 1998 CESDI 5th annual report. Department of Health, London
2. Maternal and Child Health Research Consortium 1997 CESDI 4th annual report. Department of Health, London
3. National Childbirth Trust 2001 Home birth in the United Kingdom. National Childbirth Trust, London
4. Chamberlain G, Wraight A, Crowley P 1997 Home births: the report of the 1994 confidential enquiry by the National Birthday Trust Fund. Parthenon Publishing, London
5. Annual Reports of the Registrar General for Northern Ireland.
6. Enkin M, Keirse JNC, Renfew MJ, Neilson JP 1995 A guide to effective care in pregnancy and childbirth, 2nd edn. Oxford University Press, Oxford
7. Office for National Statistics 2001 Birth statistics. Series FM1. HMSO, London
8. Dowsell T, Thornton JG, Hewison J, Lilford RJL, Raisler J, Macfarlene A 1996 Should there be a trial of home versus hospital delivery in the United Kingdom? British Medical Journal 312: 753–757
9. Olsen O, Jewell MD 2000 Home versus hospital birth (Cochrane Review). The Cochrane Library, Issue 4. Update Software, Oxford
10. Lavin JP, Stephens RJ, Miodovnik M, Barden TP 1982 Vaginal delivery in patients with a prior Caesarean section. Obstetrics and Gynecology 59: 135–148
11. Lewis G, Drife J (eds) 2001 Why mothers die 1997–1999, fifth report on confidential enquiries into maternal deaths in the United Kingdom. Royal College of Obstetricians and Gynaecologists Press, London.
12. Office for Populations, Census and Surveys 1995 Health Survey for England 1992, OPCS, London

13. Peterson S, Mockford C, Rayner M 1999 Coronary heart disease statistics. British Heart Foundation, London
14. Royal College of Obstetricians and Gynaecologists 2001 Induction of labour. Guidelines no. 9. Royal College of Obstetricians and Gynaecologists Press, London
15. British National Formulary 1997 Number 34, September 1997
16. Royal College of Obstetricians and Gynaecologists 2001 The use of electronic fetal monitoring. Guidelines no. 8. Royal College of Obstetricians and Gynaecologists Press, London
17. O'Leary JA 1992 Shoulder dystocia and birth injury: prevention and treatment. McGraw-Hill Inc, London
18. Royal College of Pathologists 1993 Guidelines for post mortem reports. Royal College of Pathologists, London
19. Gompels MJ 1998 CESDI Wessex and The Channel Islands 1997. Wessex Institute for Health Research & Development, Southampton
20. Hannah ME, Hannah WJ, Hewson SA, Hodnett ED, Saigal S, Willan AR, for the Term Breech Trial Collaborative Group 2000 Planned caesarean section versus planned vaginal birth for breech presentation at term: a randomised multicentre trial. Lancet 356: 1375–1383
21. Somerset D 2001 The term breech trial does not provide unequivocal evidence. British Medical Journal Rapid Response 8th August
22. Hofmeyer GL 2000 External cephalic version facilitation for breech presentation at term. Cochrane Database Systematic Review 2000; CD000184.
23. Royal College of Obstetricians and Gynecologists 2001 The management of breech presentation. Guideline no. 20. Royal College of Obstetricians and Gynaecologists, London
24. ALSO 1998 Advanced life support in obstetrics. The American Academy of Family Physicians
25. Nursing and Midwifery Council 2003 Standards for records and record keeping. Nursing and Midwifery Council, London

Chapter **7**

Sudden unexpected deaths in infancy

Rosie Thompson and Peter Fleming

After the 'Back to Sleep' campaign was initiated in the UK the incidence of SIDS fell dramatically by 50%.

INTRODUCTION

The enquiry into sudden unexpected deaths in infancy (SUDI) started on 1st February 1993 in two regions, South Western and Yorkshire; Trent joined later that year. In the second year of the study Northern and Wessex joined the study, which ended on 31st March 1996, covering a population of approximately 17.7 million.

The SUDI study had three linked components: a case-control study, confidential enquiries by regional assessment panels and additional pathology investigations. All three components have been published in *Sudden Unexpected Deaths in Infancy: The CESDI SUDI Studies.*[1] This chapter concentrates on the instances of suboptimal care given by professionals or by carers that panels identified throughout the 3 years of the study as possibly or probably contributing to the death of the baby.

BACKGROUND

In the 1980s, SUDIs claimed over 1000 lives each year in the UK. For some of these deaths a cause was subsequently determined, either by scrutiny of the circumstances or by autopsy. However, for the vast majority no clear cause was found: the deaths remained unexplained and were, therefore, categorized as sudden infant death syndrome (SIDS). The diagnosis is reached by exclusion, by failing to demonstrate an adequate cause of death.

A strong association between the prone-sleeping position (infants sleeping on their front) and the risk of SIDS found in the Netherlands[2] was confirmed by studies in Avon.[3] As a result, a publicity campaign was launched in an effort to heighten public awareness of this risk. In October 1991 the 'Back to Sleep' campaign was initiated in the UK and the incidence of SIDS fell dramatically by 50%.

Despite the dramatic fall in the number of deaths, the scale of the problem and our lack of understanding remain unchanged. SIDS now accounts for 20% rather than 50% of all postneonatal deaths, yet it is still the largest single group of deaths within this age group, three times higher than infant mortality from congenital heart disease. The change in sleeping position is clearly a significant factor, yet there is no medical explanation as to the causal mechanism of death resulting from using the prone-sleeping position.

In the last 50 years many studies have been conducted to find out why these deaths occur and there is broad agreement on some of the epidemiological findings. The majority of deaths occur within the first 8 months of life, with a peak around the 3rd and 4th month. It is more prevalent in males and the risk increases in winter months. SIDS occurs across the social strata, but is more prevalent in the socio-economically deprived groups. Hospital records show that many of the SIDS infants have lower birthweight and shorter gestation. Maternal factors are important; there is a strong correlation with young maternal age and higher parity, and the risk increases with multiple births.[4]

The National Advisory Body for CESDI selected sudden deaths in infancy to be the subject of one of the first detailed studies undertaken in 1993.[5] The broader category of SUDI rather than SIDS was chosen because it is often not possible to distinguish between SIDS and other unexpected deaths until the full autopsy results become available, which may not be for some weeks after the death, and even then the distinction may not be clear-cut.

DEFINITION OF SUDDEN UNEXPECTED DEATH IN INFANCY

The SUDI study comprised babies who died between 7 and 365 completed days of life (i.e. post-perinatal infant deaths). The criteria for inclusion were deaths:

- that were unexpected, and unexplained at autopsy
- occurring in the course of an acute illness that was not recognized by carers and/or by health professionals as potentially life threatening
- occurring in the course of a sudden acute illness of less than 24 hours duration
- in previously healthy infants, or after illness if intensive care had been instituted within 24 hours of its onset
- arising from a pre-existing condition that had not been previously recognized by health professionals
- resulting from any form of accident, trauma or poisoning.

CONFIDENTIAL ENQUIRY PROCESS

The structure and operation of the regional assessment panels corresponded to panels for the intrapartum-related confidential enquiries. The chairs for the panels were constant, with one or two for each region. All panel members were required to be experienced and currently active in their fields. The greatest importance was placed on confidentiality; no one involved with the case were allowed to attend. A fuller description of the confidential enquiry process is described in Chapter 1 and appeared in the CESDI 3rd annual report.[6]

The information to be considered at the panel normally included the case-control questionnaire, obstetric and midwifery notes, health visitor's (HV's) notes, general practitioner's (GP's) notes, paediatrician's notes, casualty department record, post mortem report and summary from the local case discussion.

The panel's remit was to come to a consensus view on the following:

- a short summary of the facts
- classification of the cause of death
- assessment of notable factors
- any other comments concerning the adequacy of the documentation, etc.

The assessment of the 'notable factors' was carried out by the system pioneered in Exeter.[7] A notable factor was taken to be any unusual or remarkable factor connected with a SUDI, whether or not it was relevant to the death. Each notable factor was classified according to the following questions:

- Who or what was involved?
- Was the factor relevant to the death?
- Did the factor constitute a failing in clinical management?
- Would different management have made a difference to the outcome?
- Did the factor involve a failure to recognize a problem, a failure to act appropriately or a failure to communicate?

Limitations of the enquiry

In interpreting these findings, it must be borne in mind that the panels did not have the benefit of control cases or of defined standards for good care, and that their assessments were inevitably subjective. The panel validation study[5] showed that there were sometimes inconsistencies between different panels in assessing the same cases. Some panels appeared to be harsher in their judgements than others, particularly with regard to the behaviour of carers. Assessments of professional care were more consistent, being guided by the views of the corresponding panel member on the best standards of current practice. In this context, it would have been an advantage if panel membership had included a social worker. Despite these limitations, we believe that the aggregated conclusions of expert panels on such a large number of cases provide valid guidance on where and how care might be improved.

Results of the confidential enquiries

Confidential enquiries were carried out on 417 cases, of which, 346 were recorded as SIDS and 71 as explained deaths. Suboptimal care was identified in 210 of the 346 SIDS cases and 37 of the 71 deaths that were explained (Table 7.1). The expert panels considered that 61% of SIDS and 52% of the explained deaths might have been avoided with different care. In many cases, more than one instance of suboptimal care was identified, often involving professionals and carers together. The explained deaths were more likely to have had suboptimal care by professionals, compared with the SIDS, where suboptimal care was more likely to involve the carers.

Table 7.1   Cases with suboptimal care

	SIDS		Explained deaths	
Group involved	n	%	n	%
Professionals only	23	6.6	12	16.9
Carers only	123	35.5	17	23.9
Professionals and carers	64	18.5	8	11.3
Total with suboptimal care	210	60.7	37	52.1
Total with no suboptimal care	136	39.3	34	47.9
Overall total	346	100	71	100

Table 7.2   Professionals involved in suboptimal care

	SIDS		Explained deaths	
Professional group	n = 346	%	n = 71	%
Health visitors	40	11.6	6	8.5
General practitioners	29	8.4	14	19.7
Paediatricians	34	9.8	10	14.1
Obstetricians	5	1.4	2	2.8
Hospital midwives	3	0.9	1	1.4
Community midwives	5	1.4	2	2.8
Children's nurses	0	0	2	2.8
Casualty doctors	3	0.9	1	1.4
Casualty nurses	1	0.3	0	0
CONI* nurse	1	0.3	0	0
Physiotherapist	1	0.3	0	0
Ambulance staff	0	0	1	1.4
Social workers	21	6.1	0	0

*CONI, care of the next infant

SUBOPTIMAL CARE

Suboptimal care by professionals

Table 7.2 shows the number of cases in which various professional groups delivered care that the panels considered to be suboptimal. Since most SIDS deaths occurred at home it is to be expected that the professionals most often involved would be the primary-care team, namely the HVs and GPs. Babies dying from diseases are more likely to have come to the attention of their GP or of a paediatrician, therefore, medical care came under scrutiny more often in the explained deaths group. Involvement of obstetricians as well as paediatricians reflects the increased mortality among babies with previous health problems, while involvement of social workers in cases of SIDS reflects its associations with social deprivation and with the possibility of abuse.

Suboptimal care by health visitors

Since HVs are required to see all families with new babies, they are the group most exposed to criticism when death occurs unexpectedly at home. Suboptimal care by HVs was noted in 40 (12%) cases of SIDS, 61 instances being identified in all. HVs were also criticized with regard to some of the explained deaths. Details of the instances in which panels thought that suboptimal care by the HV might have contributed to the death of the baby are given in Table 7.3.

The most frequent criticism was inadequacy of visits. This usually arose when the HV had not given extra support in a case of particular need, for example, if the baby was vulnerable or the mother immature or the home circumstances very poor. Advice might be regarded as inadequate if some aspect of the mother's care was faulty, for example, putting the baby to sleep prone, and there was no record that the HV had tried to correct her. HVs were criticized on 14 occasions for not

Table 7.3 Suboptimal care by health visitors

| | Instances | | | |
| | SIDS | | Explained deaths | |
Area of concern	$n = 346$	%	$n = 71$	%
Inadequate contact or support	21	6.1	2	2.8
Inadequate advice	16	4.6	0	0
Failure to make medical referral	10	2.9	4	5.6
Failure to monitor baby's weight	4	1.2	0	0
Failure to recognize or act on maternal depression	4	1.2	1	1.4
Failure to recognize risk of abuse	3	0.9	0	0
Poor record keeping	1	0.3	0	0
Poor communication with general practitioner	1	0.3	0	0
Poor communication with social worker	1	0.3	0	0
Total	61	17.6	7	9.9

referring the case to the GP when they should have been aware that the baby had a problem requiring medical attention; in four of these cases, the problem was urgent and led to the baby's death. Other areas attracting criticism in more than one instance were failure to weigh babies often enough, to arrange help for mothers with depression and to recognize risk of abuse.

Suboptimal care by general practitioners

Suboptimal care by GPs was identified in 29 (8%) cases of SIDS and 14 (20%) explained deaths, 60 instances being cited in all. Details are given in Table 7.4. The commonest criticism in respect of SIDS, corresponding with that of HVs, was the failure to recognize that a particular baby was vulnerable and to give adequate medical supervision. For explained deaths, the area that most frequently gave rise to concern was failure to recognize the severity of a baby's illness. GPs were also criticized on five occasions for not responding to depression in the mother, and twice for not paying sufficient attention to social problems. In four instances, the records kept by

Table 7.4 Suboptimal care by general practitioners

	Instances			
	SIDS		Explained deaths	
Area of concern	n = 346	%	n = 71	%
Failure to recognize vulnerability of baby and/ or to provide adequate medical supervision	15	4.3	0	0
Failure to recognize severity of acute illness	4	1.2	10	14.1
Failure to recognize or act on maternal depression	5	1.4	0	0
Inadequate or incorrect advice	4	1.2	0	0
Poor record keeping	4*	–	0	0
Failure to see baby when requested	2	0.6	2	2.8
Failure to appreciate social problems	1	0.3	2	2.8
Failure to recognize risk of abuse	2	0.6	0	0
Poor communication	1	0.3	1	1.4
Poor relationship with family	1	0.3	0	0
Incorrect clinical management	1	0.3	5	7.0
Total	40	11.6	20	28.2

*Based on sample only

the GP were deemed to be so poor as possibly to have contributed to the baby's death, on the grounds that another doctor seeing the baby was not sufficiently alerted to previous concerns. In many other cases, no assessment of the general practice records was possible because they were not made available to the panel. There were four criticisms for failing to see a baby when the request, in the opinion of the panel, should have received priority, and four for giving mothers advice that was incorrect or inadequate. In five of the explained deaths, the management of the final illness by the GP was thought to have been faulty.

Example 1

A 3-month-old girl was abandoned by her mother and left in the care of her father, who was unemployed, took various illegal and legal drugs and led a chaotic lifestyle. The social services department was alerted, who put the baby on the Child Protection Register. The HV visited frequently and recorded a fall-off in weight from the 50th to the 10th centile over the next few months. The baby then developed a respiratory infection and was given antibiotics, but died unexpectedly at home. No significant abnormalities were found at autopsy and the death was registered as SIDS.

The panel thought that the baby's death probably arose from low standards of care. The HV was criticized for failing to take action over the poor weight gain that she had documented.

Note: Some details have been changed to protect confidentiality, but the essential points remain.

Example 2

A 6-week-old girl developed a cough and was taken to the GP. He examined the baby and prescribed an antibiotic, and asked the HV to visit next day to check her progress. When the HV called, the mother pointed out that the baby was breathing faster than usual; she was drowsy and had been unable to take her medicine. The HV advised that she should be taken back to the surgery the next day if there was no improvement. Later that evening, the baby abruptly deteriorated and died on the way to hospital. Autopsy revealed widespread staphylococcal pneumonia.

While recognizing that staphylococcal infection may progress very rapidly, the panel thought that the HV had failed to appreciate the severity of the baby's illness at the time of her visit.

Note: Some details have been changed to protect confidentiality, but the essential points remain.

Example 3

A boy aged 3 months had been previously healthy but then began to vomit, and stopped passing faeces and urine. The vomit became green and specks of blood appeared in the nappy. The GP was called during the night but found no abnormality. The vomiting continued, and the GP was called again the next day, when he prescribed Gaviscon. Forty-eight hours after the onset of the vomiting, the baby became very ill and was taken direct to hospital. Laparotomy revealed intussusception and extensive necrosis. Despite surgery and life support the baby died.

The panel concluded that the death could have been avoided if the GP had recognized the typical features of intussusception at an earlier stage.

Note: Some details have been changed to protect confidentiality, but the essential points remain.

Example 4

A young single mother took her 3-month-old baby boy to her doctor in the morning because he felt very hot and had a skin temperature of over 40°C, was off his feeds and had sticky eyes. The doctor examined the baby briefly and prescribed eye drops. Later in the day the baby began to vomit repeatedly and became very drowsy. The mother called the practitioner and was told to come at the end of evening surgery. She took the baby straight away nevertheless, but by the time the doctor was free to see him he was limp and unresponsive. The mother was told to take him to hospital in her car; she was delayed and when she arrived the baby was dead. Autopsy showed septicaemia with adrenal haemorrhage.

The panel considered that the GP was at fault for not recognizing the severity of the baby's illness when he saw him that morning, and for not calling an ambulance when he saw him again later.

Note: Some details have been changed to protect confidentiality, but the essential points remain.

Suboptimal care by paediatricians

Panels thought that suboptimal care by paediatricians might have contributed to 34 cases (10%) of SIDS and 10 (14%) explained deaths, citing 40 and 15 instances respectively (Table 7.5). The apparently large number of criticisms of secondary care for deaths that occurred at home reflects the fact that in many cases of SIDS there is a pre-existing medical problem that contributes to the death without it being the whole cause. Failures to recognize the severity of illness preceding an explained death usually involved a less experienced

Table 7.5   Suboptimal care by paediatricians

| Area of concern | Instances | | | |
| | SIDS | | Explained deaths | |
	n = 346	%	*n* = 71	%
Poor clinical management	9	2.6	3	4.2
Failure to recognize severity of illness	1	0.3	5	7.0
Inadequate investigation	7	2.0	3	4.2
Poor discharge arrangements	2	0.6	1	1.4
Inadequate follow-up	6	1.7	0	0
Failure to take account of social background	0	0	2	2.8
Failure to recognize or act upon risk of abuse	9	2.6	0	0
Lack of leadership	3	0.9	0	0
Poor communication with general practitioner	3	0.9	1	1.4
Total	40	11.6	15	21.1

doctor who was inadequately supervised. In both SIDS and the explained group, there were criticisms for inadequate investigation, poor clinical management and unsatisfactory arrangements for discharge or follow-up. Paediatricians were criticized on nine occasions for their failure to recognize or act upon a risk of abuse. Although other health professionals may also have been involved, the paediatrician was singled out for criticism because he or she was expected to take the lead on this issue. In three cases, lack of leadership by the paediatrician was specifically mentioned. There were four criticisms of poor communication; these arose when the paediatrician had failed to discuss concerns about a vulnerable baby directly with the GP, relying instead on written reports that were delayed or not sufficiently informative.

Example 5

A baby girl was admitted to hospital at the age of 6 months because she seemed to be generally unwell. She was found to be hypoglycaemic and responded to treatment with intravenous glucose. She was sent home after 48 hours without further investigations. The parents were not advised on her feeding regime but were asked to test her blood glucose at intervals, for which equipment was provided. A few days later, they found blood glucose of 2 mmol/l in the evening and brought her back to hospital. She was normoglycaemic after a feed and was sent back home again. A week later, she was found dead in her cot at night, having apparently been normal and healthy during the day. No significant abnormalities were found at autopsy, but tests for metabolic abnormalities were incomplete. The death was registered as SIDS.

The panel thought that this baby might not have died if her recurrent hypoglycaemia had been adequately investigated and treated. The consultant paediatrician was deemed to be at fault, and the adequacy of the autopsy was also criticized.

Note: Some details have been changed to protect confidentiality, but the essential points remain.

Suboptimal care by obstetricians

It was judged that suboptimal care by obstetricians might have contributed to five cases of SIDS and to two explained deaths. In three cases, the obstetrician was held partly responsible for the vulnerability of a baby who later died from SIDS: one was the product of a multiple pregnancy induced in a young mother, another was born after unchecked premature labour, and the third was asphyxiated during breech delivery. In another instance, traumatic delivery was thought to have adversely affected a mother's attitude to her baby. Obstetricians were also criticized for poor communication, once with a mother and once with a paediatric colleague, for not heeding a family history of infant deaths, and for poor technique in resuscitating a baby.

Example 6

A mother who disliked hospitals ruptured her membranes early and was febrile by the time of delivery. A precautionary culture of the baby's blood grew *Streptococcus pyogenes* group B and treatment with intravenous antibiotics was started. However, after 48 hours the mother insisted on taking him home and was required to sign a form acknowledging that she was doing so against medical advice. The baby became unwell over the next few days and the GP visited twice, but he had not been informed of the infection. The baby steadily deteriorated and died, and at autopsy was found to have streptococcal pneumonia.

In addition to noting the mother's disregard of medical advice, the panel also criticized the paediatrician for failing to ensure adequate treatment of the baby's infection, and for failing to alert the GP to a potentially dangerous situation.

Note: Some details have been changed to protect confidentiality, but the essential points remain.

Suboptimal care by midwives

Panels criticized hospital midwives in four cases, in two for giving bad advice, in one for not paying enough attention to a mother's psychiatric problems, and in another for failing to recognize a risk of abuse. Community midwives were criticized in seven cases for nine instances of suboptimal care: in three for not providing adequate supervision, in two for not recognizing the vulnerability of the baby, in two for not making a medical referral for a baby who was unwell, in one for failure to weigh a baby who was feeding poorly, and in one for poor communication.

Suboptimal care by casualty doctors or nurses

Suboptimal care by casualty staff was thought possibly to have contributed to five deaths. Casualty doctors were criticized three times, and a casualty nurse once, for failing to get a paediatrician to see a baby that a worried mother had brought to their department. In another instance, the casualty doctor's attempt to resuscitate a baby was thought to be inadequate.

Suboptimal care by other health professionals

Children's nurses were criticized in two cases on three grounds: failure to recognize significant deterioration in a sick baby, incompetent use of a monitor and poor technique in resuscitation. There was one criticism each of a physiotherapist for advising a mother whose baby's hips had been unstable to lie him prone; of a specialist nurse, visiting under the scheme for the care of the next infant (CONI), for failing to recognize a risk of abuse; and of an ambulance man for using the wrong technique in attempting to resuscitate a collapsed baby.

Suboptimal care by social workers

In evaluating this section, it should be borne in mind that panel membership did not include a social worker, and that if it had, the number and nature of the comments might well have been different. As it was, panels thought that suboptimal care by social workers might have contributed to 21 (6%) of the cases of SIDS (Table 7.6). This proportion reflects the greater incidence of SIDS among disadvantaged families who need social-work support and the difficulties that sometimes arise in distinguishing between SIDS and deaths resulting from maltreatment. Statutory responsibility for

Table 7.6   Suboptimal care by social workers

Area of concern	Instances	
	n	%
Failure to recognize or act upon risk of abuse	15	4.3
Inadequate support for disadvantaged mother	2	0.6
Inappropriate alternative care arrangements for baby	3	0.9
Poor communication with health visitor	1	0.3
Total	21	6.1

child protection is vested primarily with social service departments, and the most frequent area of criticism was failure to recognize or act upon a risk of abuse. This usually occurred in cases where the panel suspected that death had arisen from some form of maltreatment, and where a social services department knew about the family but had not taken the appropriate preventative measures, such as holding a multi-disciplinary conference to agree a plan of protection. Social workers were also criticized for their inadequate support of two disadvantaged mothers who could not cope with their babies, and for allowing inappropriate arrangements for the alternative care of three other babies. Poor communication with the HV was also cited on one occasion.

Example 7

A fourth baby, a girl, was born to a family well known to the social services department. One of their previous children had died suddenly at the age of 3 months, and the other two were on the Child Protection Register. The HV was very concerned about standards of care and visited frequently. On two occasions, the parents said that they had had to shake the baby because she looked pale. One morning at the age of 7 weeks she was found dead in her cot. The autopsy showed no evidence of trauma and the death was registered as SIDS.

The panel thought the baby probably died as a result of poor care or maltreatment, and criticized the social worker concerned for failing to convene a multidisciplinary conference at which a plan of supervision and protection could be agreed before the baby left the maternity unit.

Note: Some details have been changed to protect confidentiality, but the essential points remain.

Contributory factors involving carers

For deaths that occur at home, it is to be expected that the behaviour of parents and other carers should come under careful scrutiny.

Table 7.7   Carers involved in contributory factors

Carer	SIDS		Explained deaths	
	$n = 346$	%	$n = 71$	%
Both parents	117	33.8	14	19.7
Mother	89	25.7	9	12.7
Father	20	5.8	0	0
Grandparents	13	3.8	1	1.4
Other relatives	3	0.9	0	0
Baby-minder	1	0.3	0	0
Total of cases involving carers	187	54.0	24	33.8

*Many cases involved more than one carer

In 187 cases (54%) of SIDS, panels identified a total of 397 factors involving parents or other carers that they thought might have contributed to the death. In many cases, more than one member of the family was implicated. Panels also noted 54 factors relating to carers in 24 (34%) of the explained deaths. The people involved are shown in Table 7.7. As would be expected, mothers, with or without their partners, were the carers most frequently involved. The relatively small number of criticisms specific to fathers reflects the infrequency with which fathers care for babies on their own. Grandparents and other relatives were sometimes involved, but there was only one instance involving a baby-minder outside the family.

Table 7.8 gives details of all the contributory factors involving carers that were identified. Some of these could be categorized under suboptimal care, for which the person concerned could fairly be held responsible, but others involved circumstances such as poverty or depression, over which the carer could have little or no control. In many cases, several different factors were noted. The factors are listed under six different headings: personal situation, social circumstances, substance abuse, infant care, sleeping arrangements and use of services. The areas incurring most frequent criticism were substance abuse and sleeping arrangements. Variation between panels was apparent here, with some but not all panels identifying as a contributory factor anything known to be associated with an increased risk of SIDS, such as smoking or prone sleeping. A more objective assessment of the prevalence and significance of these factors can be made from the case-control study.[1]

Table 7.8 Contributory factors involving carers

	Instances			
	SIDS		Explained deaths	
Area of concern	n = 346	%	n = 71	%
Personal situation (total)	26	7.5	6	8.5
Maternal depression	6	1.7	1	1.4
Other illness in mother	2	0.6	0	0
Poor hygiene	4	1.2	0	0
Poor bonding	3	0.9	0	0
Lack of support	5	1.4	1	1.4
Immaturity of mother	1	0.3	1	1.4
Learning difficulties of mother	1	0.3	0	0
Violence of father	0	0	1	1.4
Mendacity	1	0.3	0	0
Prostitution	1	0.3	0	0
Poor command of English	0	0	1	1.4
Mother absent from home	0	0	1	1.4
Mother abused in childhood	2	0.6	0	0
Social circumstances (total)	21	6.1	3	4.2
Poverty	8	2.3	2	2.8
Disorganized household	10	2.9	0	0
Travelling family	1	0.3	1	1.4
Mother in prison	1	0.3	0	0
Father in prison	1	0.3	0	0
Substance abuse (total)	137	39.6	14	19.7
Cigarettes	100	28.9	8	11.3
Alcohol	13	3.8	4	5.6
Illegal drugs	24	6.9	2	2.8
Infant care (total)	45	13.0	7	9.9
Incorrect feeding	7	2.0	2	2.8
Inadequate supervision of baby	7	2.0	4	5.6
Suspected abuse	8	2.3	0	0
Carer under influence of alcohol	13	3.8	0	0
Generally poor standards	10	2.9	1	1.4
Sleeping arrangements (total)	137	39.6	6	8.5
Inappropriate place	12	3.5	0	0
Use of unsafe cot or bunk-bed	0	0	3	4.2
Settee shared with adult	6	1.7	0	0
Bed sharing under influence of alcohol	13	3.8	0	0
Other bed sharing	19	5.5	1	1.4
Use of soft pillow	5	1.4	0	0

(continued)

Table 7.8   continued

| Area of concern | Instances | | | |
| | SIDS | | Explained deaths | |
	$n = 346$	%	$n = 71$	%
Placing baby prone	31	9.0	1	1.4
Overwrapping	29	8.4	0	0
Keeping baby too warm	16	4.6	1	1.4
Use of electric blanket	1	0.3	0	0
Leaving fire burning near baby all night	4	1.2	0	0
Not keeping baby warm enough	1	0.3	0	0
Use of services (total)	31	9.0	15	21.1
Late booking at antenatal clinic	5	1.4	2	2.8
Refusal to use services or accept advice	15	4.3	2	2.8
Failure to give medication or other treatment	2	0.6	1	1.4
Failure to recognize illness or seek advice	8	2.3	7	9.9
Refusal of hospital admission for baby	0	0	1	1.4
Taking baby out of hospital against advice	0	0	1	1.4
Incorrect resuscitation	1	0.3	1	1.4

Personal and social circumstances

Most of the aspects of the mother's personal situation that panels thought might possibly have contributed to the death of her baby, such as depression and lack of support, were factors for which she could not be held responsible. Social circumstances were also thought to have played a part in several deaths, in particular when the family was oppressed by poverty, or followed a chaotic lifestyle.

Substance abuse

Smoking, identified in previous studies as conferring an increased risk of SIDS, was noted by panels in 100 instances, much more than for any other factor. Use of illegal drugs was cited 24 times, and excessive consumption of alcohol 13 times. Several parents were criticized for abuse of all three types of substance. In addition, 13 carers were held possibly to have been responsible for the deaths by being under the influence of alcohol whilst caring for the baby.

Example 8

A 30-year-old mother looked after her four children without support, her partner having left her soon after the birth of the youngest. She was on treatment for chronic arthritis, anxiety and depression, and was prone to the abuse of alcohol and other drugs. Her flat was burgled, so she went to stay with her mother, with whom she had a stormy relationship, in very cramped accommodation. The two women smoked a total of about 40 cigarettes a day. Her fourth baby, a boy, had been asphyxiated at birth and was slow in his development. When 3 months old, he became unwell and would not feed, and was found dead in his cot in the early evening. No abnormalities were found at autopsy and the death was registered as SIDS.

The panel thought that the multiplicity of problems besetting this mother must have contributed to the death of her baby.

Note: Some details have been changed to protect confidentiality, but the essential points remain.

Infant care and sleeping arrangements

Other areas of poor infant care were inadequate supervision and incorrect feeding, usually the introduction of solids too early. In eight cases of SIDS, child abuse was raised as a possible contributory factor. With regard to sleeping arrangements, the commonest criticisms were laying the baby prone (31 instances) and over-wrapping (28 instances), both of which recent studies had shown to bring an increased risk of SIDS. There were also 16 criticisms for keeping the baby too warm in contrast to only one for not keeping the baby warm enough. Panels varied in their judgements on bed sharing, reflecting current uncertainties on the issue. Sharing a bed with an intoxicated adult, or sleeping together on a settee, were usually regarded as hazardous, being cited in 13 and six cases respectively, while bed sharing in the absence of these particular hazards was thought to be a possible contributory factor in 19 other cases. Other places regarded as inappropriate for a baby to sleep were the floor, on sofas, on full-sized beds, or in car seats. It is a tragic irony that at least three parents had transferred their babies to such places because of the publicity given to the alleged risk from cot mattresses, later shown to be unfounded.[4] Two of the explained deaths arose when a baby was accidentally hung after slipping under the horizontal bar of a bunk-bed designed for an older child, and a third baby died when a faulty cot collapsed. Parents were criticized on five occasions for leaving their baby to sleep close to coke or gas fires. Soft pillows and an electric blanket were also seen as potential sources of danger.

Example 9

A boy aged 3 months had oral thrush, a nappy rash and a mild respiratory infection for which he was taking antibiotics. His parents went out to a party leaving him in the care of a baby sitter. They came home just after midnight, having drunk a lot of alcohol, and put the baby down to sleep in his cot beside their bed as usual. They woke at 8.00 am to find the baby dead, lying in their bed and totally covered by the duvet. They could not remember what had happened during the night, but thought they had probably taken the baby into their bed for a feed and then fallen asleep. No significant abnormalities were found at autopsy and the death was registered as SIDS.

The panel thought that the baby's death resulted from sharing a bed with parents who were intoxicated.

Note: Some details have been changed to protect confidentiality, but the essential points remain.

Example 10

A 6-month-old boy with a history of wheezing became chesty and unwell. Both parents used to smoke constantly in the presence of the baby, despite advice from the HV. The mother was depressed, and the father, who was unemployed, took most of the decisions and was adverse to anyone in authority. The GP came to see the baby and advised admission to hospital. This was refused, as was another attempt at persuasion by the HV when she called later. Next morning, the baby was found dead in his cot. The autopsy showed extensive bronchiolitis and pneumonia.

The panel thought that the death might have been avoided if the parents had not refused to allow the baby to go into hospital. In addition, their heavy smoking was thought to have contributed to the illness.

Note: Some details have been changed to protect confidentiality, but the essential points remain.

Use of services

Several families were criticized for an apparent aversion to seeking or taking advice about the health of their babies. The most extreme instances were a mother who insisted on taking her baby out of hospital when he was in the early stages of an infection that proved fatal, and a father who refused to let his sick baby be admitted for hospital care. In seven cases very late booking for antenatal care was thought to have contributed to subsequent death. In eight cases of

SIDS and seven of explained death, panels thought that parents had failed to appreciate the severity of their baby's illness and had not sought vital help. In three other instances, parents did seek advice but then failed to give the treatment prescribed.

Example 11

A girl born 7 weeks prematurely made good progress while in hospital, but the HV found it difficult to obtain access to see her once she had gone home. One morning when she was 4 months old, her grandmother found her seriously ill and took her straight to hospital, but she died a few hours later. The story emerged that she had been unwell for 3 days, crying incessantly and feeding poorly. She then became very hot and drowsy. When her grandmother happened to call, she found the baby unresponsive, with wandering eyes and stiff limbs. The parents said they had not contacted the GP, as they disliked his manner.

Autopsy revealed cerebral oedema and encephalopathy, thought to be of viral origin. The panel concluded that this baby might not have died if the parents had made proper use of the services.

Note: Some details have been changed to protect confidentiality, but the essential points remain.

Carers other than mothers

Fathers and other relatives were criticized for much the same reasons as the mothers. In addition, three fathers were thought to have contributed to the death of a baby by their failure to support their partner, and two grandparents by damaging their daughter's capacity as a mother through their abuse of her as a child. The one criticism of a baby-minder was for failure to provide adequate supervision.

Inadequate resources

Panels identified 14 instances in which inadequate resources were thought to have contributed to SIDS, but only one instance involving an explained death (Table 7.9). Ten related to the material circumstances of the family, usually the adequacy of accommodation. Of those that related to the health service, there were three criticisms for the absence of cover for a HV who was off sick, and two for the lack of facilities for paediatric intensive care. The latter deficiency has since been officially acknowledged and is being addressed on a national basis.

Table 7.9   Inadequate resources

Resource	SIDS		Explained deaths	
	$n = 346$	%	$n = 71$	%
Poor accommodation	9	2.6	0	0
Poor heating	1	0.3	0	0
Lack of cover for health visitor	3	0.9	0	0
Lack of facilities for paediatric intensive care	1	0.3	1	1.4
Total of cases involving carers	14	4.0	1	1.4

CONCLUSIONS AND RECOMMENDATIONS

Many of the suboptimal factors identified in these confidential enquiries were around professionals failing to recognize serious illness in babies. This was particularly noticeable amongst GPs. It is important that all healthcare professionals are aware of the risk factors and reinforce the key messages to parents and carers.

Key recommendations

Factors for healthcare professionals to note

The factors given below are likely to be amenable to change by advice from healthcare professionals.

Encourage:

- supine sleeping position for infants
- placing the infant in the cot in the 'feet to foot' position
- sharing a room with the baby for the first 6 months.

Discourage:

- sleeping with the infant on a sofa, settee or arm chair
- bed sharing when parents are tired or have taken drugs to help sleep
- heavy wrapping and high room temperature
- the use of pillows, duvets or loose bedding (particularly if there is a risk of inadvertent head covering).

The following factors may be amenable to modification by advice from healthcare professionals, but involve a change in parental behaviour.

Encourage:

- immunization.

Discourage:

- exposure of pregnant women and infants to cigarette smoke
- bed sharing by parents who have recently consumed alcohol or illicit drugs.

The factors given below, whilst being potentially amenable to change, will require the development of a strategy to achieve a significant change in parental behaviour:

- Maternal smoking during pregnancy
- Bed sharing and smoking
- Parental alcohol or other drug abuse.

The following factors may alert healthcare professionals to the special needs of the family:

- Low maternal age
- High maternal parity (particularly if mother under 27 years)
- Low income
- Maternal smoking during pregnancy
- Smoking in the home
- Poor or crowded housing
- Single unsupported mother
- Baby of low birth weight; short gestation or multiple birth
- Baby with congenital anomaly
- Recent move of house (especially during the year before the birth) (three of the first four factors are present in 8% of the population in general, but in over 40% of SIDS families).

Whilst there is no direct evidence that improvement of social conditions decreases the risk of SIDS, the strong association of socio-economic deprivation and poor housing with SIDS should encourage healthcare professionals to work with colleagues in social services to try to improve housing conditions for such families whenever possible.

The acute factors given below may signify transient increased risk and alert family or healthcare professionals to the need for close observation or possible treatment:

- A high 'Baby Check' score
- A history of an apparent life-threatening event.

Factors for parents to note

Whilst it is not possible to guarantee that any baby will not be a victim of SIDS, following certain simple guidelines can substantially reduce the risk:

- Place your baby to sleep on his/her back, not the front or side.

- Place your baby on a clean, dry mattress. Use lightweight blankets and clothing. Avoid the use of duvets, quilts, pillows, cushions or beanbags. Check your baby to ensure that he/she does not feel too hot or too cold.

- Place your baby to sleep so that his/her feet are close to the foot of the cot ('feet to foot') with the bedding securely tucked in and no higher than the baby's chin.

- Never sleep with your baby on a sofa, settee or armchair. If you cuddle or feed your baby on a sofa, settee or armchair ensure you do not fall asleep with him/her.

- If possible, place your baby's cot in the same room as your bed.

Whilst it is safe to take your baby into bed with you to feed or for comfort, there are certain circumstances, especially in the first 4 months of life, when it is important to place him/her back in the cot before you go to sleep. These include:

- if you or your partner smoke
- if you or your partner have recently consumed alcohol
- if you or your partner have recently taken drugs which make you sleep more heavily
- if you or your partner are extremely tired.

Unlike cots, adult beds and bunk beds are not designed to meet safety standards for infants. Bunk beds pose particular risks of injury to young infants who can slip under the side safety bar and be strangled.

If you plan to sleep with your baby, make sure the baby's head cannot become covered by bedding. Keep the baby away from the pillows, use lightweight blankets rather than adult bed covers (e.g. duvets), and place your baby in a position where there is no risk of falling out of the bed.

Do not smoke during pregnancy or go into a room in which others are smoking. If you cannot completely stop, then cut down as much as possible. Do not smoke in any room in which young infants ever go. Keep your baby out of rooms in which people smoke (in other words maintain a 'smoke-free zone' around yourself whilst pregnant, and around your baby after he/she is born).

Finally, if your baby is unwell, particularly if he/she has a temperature, has any difficulty breathing, or is less responsive than usual, seek medical help promptly.

ACKNOWLEDGEMENTS

Dr Chris Bacon, Consultant Paediatrician, Yorkshire Region and Dr John Tripp, Consultant Senior Lecturer in Child Health, Royal Devon & Exeter Hospital, South Western Region, authors of Chapter 5 Results of the Confidential Enquiries in Sudden Unexpected Deaths in Infancy: The CESDI SUDI Study that has been abridged for this chapter.

The Stationery Office for kind permission to present findings from the publication *Sudden Unexpected Deaths in Infancy: The CESDI SUDI Studies*.

References

1. Fleming P (ed.) 2000 Sudden unexpected deaths in infancy: The CESDI SUDI Studies 1993–1996. The Stationery Office, London
2. De Jonge GA, Engelberts AC, Koomen-Liefting AJ, Kostense P 1989 Cot death and prone sleeping position in the Netherlands. British Medical Journal 298: 72–76
3. Wigfield RE, Fleming PJ, Berry PJ, Rudd PT, Golding J 1992 Can the fall in Avon's sudden infant death rate be explained by the observed sleeping position changes? British Medical Journal 304: 282–283
4. Hoffman HJ, Hunter JC, Ellish NJ, Janerich DT, Goldberg J 1988 Adverse reproductive factors and the sudden infant death syndrome. In: Harper RM, Hoffman HJ (eds). Sudden infant death syndrome. Risk factors and basic mechanisms. PMA Publishing, New York
5. Maternal and Child Health Research Consortium 1995 CESDI 2nd annual report. Department of Health, London
6. Maternal and Child Health Research Consortium 1996 CESDI 3rd annual report. Department of Health, London
7. Tripp JH. Exeter system (personal communication)

Chapter 8

Using the confidential enquiries to change practice

Judith Rankin, Judith Bush, Tricia Cresswell, Ruth Bell, Marjorie Renwick and Martin Ward Platt

It's very, very, very challenging because you pick over the bones very carefully in the enquiry and you go away and it raises all sorts of questions about what you're actually doing in your practice.
(Northern CESDI panel member)

INTRODUCTION

The purpose of the confidential enquiries in England and Wales is to generate change in practice to improve patient outcomes. To do this, they pool information on rare adverse outcomes (deaths) in relation to specific areas of health care, and aggregate it to produce reports.

Yet this is not self-evidently the most effective way to change practice. Although confidential enquiries have been established nationally, i.e. the Confidential Enquiries into Maternal Deaths (CEMD), the National Confidential Enquiry into Perioperative Deaths (NCEPOD) and, more recently, the Confidential Inquiry into Suicides and Homicides (CISH), it is only the Confidential Enquiries into Stillbirths and Deaths in Infancy (CESDI) that has functioned locally as well as having a national dimension.[1] This chapter addresses two main questions: does this local dimension add value to the process of confidential enquiry, and is it more effective in generating change than the other national enquiries?

This chapter attempts to define more closely the value of engaging in the confidential enquiry panel process for CESDI to the individual participants, and to the departments from which they come. This chapter describes some findings from a recent report[2] that provides evidence of the ways in which practice can be altered, and we demonstrate how change can be driven. The report suggest that if changes in practice are genuinely desired, more attention has to be given to the possibilities inherent in confidential enquiry panels, and due regard given to the power of local ownership of the enquiry process.

BACKGROUND

As previously mentioned, the CESDI was established in 1992 by the Department of Health to improve understanding of how the risks of death in late fetal life and infancy might be reduced, by specifically attempting to identify where suboptimal clinical care might have contributed to a poor outcome.[3] It had two main components:

1. A notification process (the rapid report form) for all deaths occurring between 20 weeks' gestation and 1 year of life. This contained considerably more detail than is available on death or stillbirth registration regarding classification of factors related to the death.

2. A rolling programme of confidential enquiries into subsets of the deaths which is delivered on a regional basis and coordinated nationally.

In the North of England in 1981, the Northern Regional Perinatal Mortality Survey (PMS) was established as a collaborative exercise between all the health districts in the former Northern NHS region, with the aim of studying perinatal mortality and its causes.[4] From 1993, the Regional Maternity Survey Office (RMSO), which runs the perinatal mortality survey and several other related surveys, also delivered the regional coordination function for the national CESDI. The same notification route was, therefore, used both for CESDI and for ascertaining deaths for PMS.

The methodology used for the confidential enquiries is detailed in other chapters. However, it is worth emphasizing that the CESDI process has become more sophisticated over time, with improvement made to the structure of the panel reporting process and greater clarity about the definition of suboptimal care. The more recent enquiries have used review of cases by other regions in an attempt to improve consistency,[5] and the national CESDI diabetic pregnancy enquiry, starting in 2003, measures care against explicit, agreed standards.

In the Northern CESDI region, in line with national directives, panels have been held on:

- intrapartum-related deaths in babies over 1.5 kg
- 1 in 10 sample of all deaths in babies over 1 kg
- all deaths of babies over 4 kg
- sudden unexpected deaths in infancy (deaths and control living babies/infants)
- deaths of babies born at 27/28 weeks' gestation (and living controls).

In addition, the Northern region has a longstanding audit of diabetic pregnancy administered through the RMSO.[6] In 1999, three confidential enquiry panels were held to investigate cases where the outcome was a perinatal or infant death.[7] In 2002, five panels were held to consider the quality of care in diabetic pregnancy with all outcomes. These panels have acted as a pilot for the national enquiry process mentioned before.

Panel membership is variable depending on the topic of enquiry but includes at least four experienced clinicians from the following specialties: midwifery, obstetrics, neonatal nursing, neonatology, paediatrics and pathology. For the diabetic pregnancy panels, diabetologists and diabetes specialist nurses were added and for the 27/28 week panels, health visitors and general practitioners. In the Northern region the decision was made to have a limited number of individuals acting as chairs, in order to standardize the running of the panels. Only six individuals have acted in this capacity over the 10 years, with the majority of panels being chaired by the former Clinical Director or the Director of the RMSO.

CESDI has acknowledged that the regional panels may be fulfilling an important educational role.[8] A report on the local enquiry in this region into perinatal deaths in babies weighing more than 4 kg in pregnancies complicated by diabetes, stated that panel participants 'found the discussion in a multi-disciplinary panel a stimulating learning environment.'[6] Anecdotally, other panel members have commented on how useful and important they have found participating in the confidential enquiry process. However, the educational effects and the perceived value of participating in confidential enquiry panels has not so far been formally studied.

The impact of other confidential enquiries has also been evaluated. In a questionnaire survey of anaesthetists designed to examine the impact of the National Confidential Enquiry into Perioperative Deaths (NCEPOD) on clinical practice, 74% of respondents said their personal clinical practice had been influenced, while 80% said that local guidelines or protocols were influenced by NCEPOD recommendations, as were negotiations to improve essential services, staff and equipment.[9] A telephone survey of awareness of the key recommendations from the *Report on Confidential Enquiries into Maternal Deaths in the UK 1994–96*[10] among obstetric and midwifery staff, found that 65% of respondents had read at least some of the report and that a median of three out of 18 key recommendations were recalled, but how far this report impacted on practice was not ascertained.

We, therefore, set out to discover the ways in which participating in confidential enquiry panels may have influenced professional practice among the various disciplines of medical, nursing and midwifery staff who had served on CESDI panels in the North of England.

STUDY

In total, 18 health professionals who had served on confidential enquiry panels were interviewed, with representatives from each of the professional groups involved in the panels: nursing and midwifery staff (four), obstetricians (six), paediatricians (six, including three neonatologists) and diabetologists (two). Seven had taken part in from one to four panels and 11 had taken part in five or more. The length of time over which any participant had been involved in confidential enquiry panels ranged from 1–10 years or more. Three participants had chaired panels. This yielded a rich set of qualitative data, the most important aspects of which are described below.

PURPOSE OF THE PANELS

In the view of the participants, the purpose of confidential enquiry panels is multilayered, encompassing both a technique for assessing care and also the learning element associated with attending such panels:

> *CESDI's view is that information will come out which will allow people to look at processes and in particular processes that result in poor outcomes, and therefore hope to change those processes so you get*

better outcomes and that is everybody's purpose. The people sitting on the panel, there's also the knowledge that you gain from doing it, and seeing how other units do things means that you have a much wider base of information on which to change your own practice.
(Consultant paediatrician, more than 10 panels)

Participants emphasized both the assessment of care (i.e. finding out what had gone wrong and identifying substandard care), and the value of doing this in a multidisciplinary, non-blaming, anonymous context with individuals who had not been directly involved in the cases being assessed, but who had experience in relevant fields of care. The ultimate aim was viewed as improving practice:

... trying to foster a sort of non blame kind of culture by measuring the fact that the cases were anonymised but yet it could be fed back nationally about the reasons why these things happen in order to try and get people to think about how their care is organised within the unit. What their deficiencies are, whether those are organisational deficiencies, whether they're training deficiencies or what, it is about things that happen that result in an adverse outcome.
(Consultant obstetrician, more than 10 panels)

The educational value was seen both in terms of learning from bad outcomes and errors in care, and from the mix of views of other disciplines represented on the panels:

It's a learning experience and it's also a very supportive environment. I have found that people are sort of saying, oh we wouldn't do it that way. There's an interaction between the panelists which is very good. And at the end of it I don't think there's any one that I have ever been involved with where I haven't come away thinking oh I will remember that or do that differently or we need to look at it, which is why I am really keen to do them. Because you can tell, because I've found them personally that's one of the ways I learn. I'd far rather do that than go and sit in a meeting or a conference or something. I think I take away from these things far more than sort of passive learning.
(Consultant obstetrician, several panels)

Attendance at panels was valued by different professionals and was seen as worth prioritizing, though it was not always easy:

It is a problem ... one of the reasons why I have only attended a couple is because of the time constraints. I see no way around it though I do actually believe in the concept of these confidential enquiries and if it's at all possible I like to cooperate with them but time is the major constraint.
(Consultant obstetrician, two panels)

It was a very interesting meeting so even if it maybe appeared lengthy in terms of what we produced we then discussed around the points so, you know, it was a worthwhile productive day.
(Diabetic nurse specialist, one panel)

It is perhaps a further indication of the value attached to attending panels that members considered it worthwhile to put in the considerable quantity of preparatory work that is necessary if the panel is to work effectively:

I actually did a very, very detailed review of all four sets of notes on the first occasion and em ..., you know, some of the notes were two volumes and it was a huge amount of work. It couldn't conceivably have been done during the morning.
(Consultant diabetologist, two panels)

Around half of the participants felt that particular insight and expertise had been missing from some of the panels they had attended and that representatives from particular professional or specialty groups should have been invited to attend. Consultants and diabetic nurse specialists felt that dieticians and midwives would have provided important expertise for panels involving pregnancies affected by diabetes. Several participants felt that anaesthetists should have been invited. Junior doctors were also viewed as a group who would benefit from attending panels for learning purposes. A small number of participants felt that patients and the medical staff involved in the cases discussed could also provide important insights, although this would be contrary to the confidential nature of the enquiries. One participant felt that the opinion of clinicians working outside of the region would be of benefit in terms of comparing practice. However, there was also caution about the need to restrict panel group size.

GROUP DYNAMICS: ACHIEVING CONSENSUS

All participants felt that the quality of the discussion at most of the panel meetings they had attended had been good in terms of equality of participation and freedom to express ideas. With a small number of exceptions, the chairing of the meetings was viewed as having been very effective in enabling people to participate and speak equally. The atmosphere was often described as 'friendly' and 'supportive' with a good level of interaction between participants:

I think probably the first one of these was quite a long time ago and initially I was pleasantly surprised by the multidisciplinary nature of the meeting and by the willingness of non-consultant medical staff and their willingness to contribute in a non-intimidated fashion. (Consultant paediatrician, many panels)

However, participants stated the standard of discussion had varied between the panels they had attended. In some panels, certain individuals had tried to dominate the discussion, although the chairs had often been successful in terms of handling this and encouraging other people to speak.

IMPACT ON PERSONAL PRACTICE

The multidisciplinary and multihospital nature of panels meant that panelists were able to reflect upon their practice and compare procedures and standards in their own department, both with those of the cases being discussed in the meeting and with other panelists. Taking part in panels was also felt to 'increase awareness' of standards of care:

It's very, very, very challenging because you pick over the bones very carefully in the enquiry and you go away and it raises all sorts of questions about what you're actually doing in your practice. So it's very helpful I think. It gives you a fair amount of enthusiasm to try to, to look with a sort of outside perspective and say, how's it going, are we doing better than these people are doing? What are they doing well that we can borrow, all of that sort of stuff. So in that sense it has actually changed our practice ... I think we all had a document with the standards in the back but when you're measuring things against them through a whole half day you become really quite aware of things ... it was a very good piece of reflective practice if you like, it produced a reflective process which was I think very helpful. (Consultant diabetologist, two panels)

Learning impacts occurred in a variety of different contexts:

... just by reading through the notes you can get information from the layout. Wow that's a good way of doing it or that's a very bad way of doing it. So you learn from just the way the records are kept. You learn from the information that was there in terms of how people conduct themselves and again, both good things you want to emulate and things you want to avoid. And then there were, at times when you felt that the information you had gathered was so poor that something needed to be done about it. In other words, a practice that was unacceptable ... and they needed to understand that their practice

needed to change. So you've got the global thing, you've got the personal thing and then you've got another, sort of a direct effect too. So it's very complex.
(Consultant paediatrician, more than 10 panels)

Organizational learning was highlighted by many participants. The main impact associated with taking part in panels was a heightened awareness of the importance of good documentation, and the need for clinical notes to be written in a clear and accessible way so that other people can follow the train of thought. In some cases this had led to departments introducing new forms. Participants had also noticed the importance of including the grades of relevant members of staff on notes and acknowledging personal accountability for documentation:

I thought it was a very good learning experience because when you're actually looking after someone yourself, you know, you document as much as you can, you don't realise some of the obvious things that maybe you know but you don't actually write down.
(Diabetes nurse specialist, one panel)

Some participants felt that taking part in panels had had an important impact in terms of increasing their awareness of personal accountability in providing care and in decision making, and the importance of effective communication:

(Panels make me reflect on) organisational things really. The way the unit is structured. You can see that there's a problem developing and you think well actually if personnel got involved at that stage rather than waiting to come in at that stage you could have probably dealt with these better.
(Consultant obstetrician, several panels)

CLINICAL KNOWLEDGE

There seemed to be a degree of clinical learning from the expertise of other panelists at the meetings, although this was less than the learning related to organizational issues:

I think it has been educational. I mean obviously you know obstetrics is what I am interested in, it's what I've been trained in, and I would like to think I am reasonably up on that. But there is quite a lot of neonatal things you know. I've never have any, some obstetricians do, I never did do any neonatology in my training and therefore that's

very interesting to me to hear the neonatologist talk about what they do, aspects of resuscitation and what they do in relation to what we do, how what we do may impinge upon you know what they need to know and so on. And also from a pathology point of view the influence from (name) has been very valuable you know.
(Consultant obstetrician, more than 10 panels)

Some participants felt taking part in a panel was a far more effective learning environment than many other examples of postgraduate and training programmes:

I think this has been some of the most useful personal postgraduate, if you want to call it that, activity I have done over the last seven or eight years. I've never been to a CESDI panel and come away thinking that was a waste of time. I've come out of every one having had an opportunity to reflect, having had an opportunity to, in some ways, sympathise with the people that were dealing with the problems in some ways, criticise in a very structured and supportive way the way cases were handled.
(Consultant obstetrician, several panels)

At the time I remember saying to some of the midwives here this is more productive in terms of updating you than any study day you can do about aromatherapy or baby massage … because it made you read up on the references otherwise you'd look a right fool. Sitting there saying well actually you know I don't think we should have done that and the evidence would have indicated that you know you were completely wrong with your opinions so it made you read the kind of case. So I thought in fact I wrote to the ENB as it was at the time and said that these appearances because that's what they were really at these confidential enquiries should be accredited in terms of updating and they agreed.
(Nurse manager, several panels)

However, while acknowledging the value of reflection, one participant was less sure about any impact on personal practice as they felt there were no objective measurement of such change:

I mean the specific things are notes, communication with parents, what consultants have put in the notes, decision making, I mean it just generally makes me reflect on what I do for a few weeks. Whether it's changed my practice or not although I'd like to think it has but again there's no objective measure of it.
(Consultant paediatrician, six panels)

Around two-thirds of participants had discussed their participation in enquiry panels with colleagues. Most had done this informally, via discussions and conversations. A small number of participants had fed back formally via presentations and meetings. Some of the specialist nurses and midwives who took part in the study described how they had used the presentation skills developed for the enquiry panels to take part in such meetings. All participants stated that they would encourage a colleague to take part in a confidential enquiry panel as the educative value of taking part was considered to be high. Importantly, this suggests both that the educational value was not confined to the participants, and that participation helped some individuals with aspects of personal and professional development in unpredictable ways.

CLINICAL FUNCTION WITHIN DEPARTMENTS

Over half of the participants stated that taking part in a confidential enquiry panel had had an impact on practice in their department. Sometimes the influence was direct and immediate:

I have been part of a panel where at the morning coffee break a participant went off, phoned his own unit and said change our way of doing this. Right. Instant feedback. 'I've just done a CESDI panel and what we've been doing for years is wrong we need to change it right.' So impact, right. So we were all well impressed with that.
(Consultant obstetrician, several panels)

More commonly, taking part in a panel was one of several 'influences' that had led to changes being introduced in a department. Several participants also described how taking part in a panel had 'reinforced' the importance of certain aspects of care without necessarily bringing about direct changes:

Intrapartum care. I feel that, you know, in reinforcing things like, especially with the junior doctors and making sure that there's adequate senior cover and things like that. So reinforcement rather than make changes in practice but ensuring that we do, people do follow the protocols that we have established which are along the national guidance, the NICE guidelines and RCOG guidelines and that deviations are only undertaken at consultant level, not other people taking short cuts. And it's all documented.
(Consultant obstetrician, several panels)

The main impacts at department level were related to standards of documentation and introducing new forms or changing existing ones:

Well it certainly heightened record keeping. And that had sort of been on my mind for quite a while, but what it did do it pushed me into saying, right, we've actually now made a form that matches the pregnancy but it's for pre-conception. It's kept at the Diabetes Centre. And then when the patient becomes pregnant and we've had all this input, there's a copy taken and it goes into the notes. So we've managed to do that. I actually got down to doing it, not just by myself, I did it with the consultant and another nurse but we actually managed to do it. (Diabetic nurse specialist, one panel)

We revamped a form that we use here after I'd seen one in somebody else's pile (of notes). I think it was a fluid balance summary sheet. (Nurse specialist, several panels)

Some participants had applied the skills developed to assess care in the context of confidential enquiry panels, and lessons learned, to assessing standards of care and organization of their own departments.

Those clinicians who took part in the study and who were also involved in teaching felt that taking part in panels had influenced practices relating to undergraduate teaching and training of junior doctors in their departments. There was now a conscious move towards familiarizing junior staff with the CESDI approach for assessing care, involving them in discussions of case studies, developing skills in being able to assess what went wrong and why, and learning the importance of good documentation. Sometimes junior members of staff had been invited to participate in a CESDI type of panel when they had been involved with a poor outcome, although some were not comfortable taking part in such a process:

Firstly we always try and ensure that when we're having our perinatal mortality meetings that the junior staff are aware of how that then contributes to the survey and to CESDI. We try and classify each case on CESDI lines. But sometimes it's difficult to talk about, there may be sensitivities and we actually stopped doing that because it's not helpful. And we try and ensure that when there's been a CESDI report we actually present it and ensure that everyone knows what the recommendations are and try and ensure we translate them into our guidelines and practice. And then obviously we set up the training sessions, the joint training sessions for paediatricians and obstetricians which was well received, good feedback ... (we need to get) junior staff appreciating what it's like to look at a set of notes fourteen months down the line. What were you thinking, because you've not recorded what you were thinking, what you were

planning. And we've got to find a way of translating that so that we can help them to appreciate the value of good documentation.
(Consultant obstetrician, several panels)

Only a small number of participants felt that there had been no significant impact on departmental practice as a result of their taking part in a panel:

... there might be certain points that you might change within a guideline ... but I've not come out of a panel and thought we should change supervision because of the panels. Rather than we need more supervision because we need it generally.
(Consultant obstetrician, several panels)

However, several others talked about the constraints they faced (often time related), which had restricted the potential impacts of taking part in panels:

It gives you a fair amount of enthusiasm to try to look with a sort of outside perspective and say, how's it going, are we doing better than these people are doing, what are they doing well that we can borrow, all of that sort of stuff. So in that sense it has actually changed our practice. We've given ourselves all sorts of good resolutions which have failed to be implemented but that's largely about all of us being much more busy than we'd like to be ... we wanted to make our group more cohesive and meet more often, the main obstacle to that has been nothing to do with CESDI, it's simply been that I'm trying to have too many hats on at the moment.
(Consultant diabetologist, two panels)

NETWORKING

Panels gave participants the opportunity to network and meet with colleagues from other specialties, other hospitals and other disciplines; this was highly valued:

I think it's very valuable because you can put a face to a name. It helps for future networking. If you're going to refer a patient in future you've got some idea of who it is you're talking to. So I think it's very valuable.
(Consultant obstetrician, several panels)

I mean it's a great help with communications in the region, you know, I mean if any of our babies go to [unit x] or [unit y], I've actually met some of their medical staff, nursing staff, you know, and that has to be positive.
(Specialist nurse, six panels)

KEY MESSAGES

The participants in this study were enthusiastic about confidential enquiry panels in terms of their own learning, the impacts on their departments, their practice and that of their colleagues, and a number of other less tangible benefits that could not have been predicted in advance. They were able to cite concrete examples of change, and took evident pride in their part in driving change.

This is direct evidence of the value of locally based panels in changing practice in that locality: in this case, the former Northern Region. It contrasts with the perceptions of the CESDI reports, which, although well regarded, are not seen as being capable of driving change or generating the passion and motivation that participation in the panels can achieve.

For quality and safety to improve, it is well recognized that 'flat' structures, teams rather than hierarchies, and interprofessional respect are pivotal.[11] One of the clear benefits of panel participation is the opportunity to develop interprofessional respect, and to do so in a non-hierarchical setting where the quest for the 'truth' in each CESDI case is a team effort. Participants evidently realized and valued this effect, and it is likely to have permeated their departments cumulatively over the time span of the CESDI enterprise.

One of the disadvantages of the CESDI approach is its emphasis on deficient practice in relation to adverse outcomes. Yet participants often recognize that there are aspects of high-quality practice to be found even in cases where the outcome was a death, and it is a source of frustration that there is no way of capturing and celebrating the good things. However, it is possible to frame a confidential enquiry in such a way that the positives as well as the negatives are captured, and this approach has been used in an evaluation of neonatal nurse practitioners undertaken in the North of England.[12] It follows that there is still potential to develop the confidential enquiry process further, with the possibility of increasing its value even more for the participants.

Confidential enquiries, when run in the CESDI fashion, can be a powerful tool both to educate and to drive change through the experiences of the participants on the panels. Over 30 years ago the environmental movement gave the world the idea of 'think global, act local': it would seem that this applies just as strongly to the effectiveness of confidential enquiry.

ACKNOWLEDGEMENTS

We are very grateful to all the staff for taking the time to be interviewed. We thank Dr Chris Wright for advice, and Terry Lisle, Emma Hutchinson and Carole Frazer for secretarial support. Dr Judith Bush was supported by funds from the Regional Maternity Surveys Office.

References

1. Grimley Evans J 2000 Review of confidential enquiries for the National Institute for Clinical Excellence. National Institute for Clinical Excellence, London
2. Rankin J, Bush J, Cresswell P, Bell R, Renwick M 2003 A qualitative study of the impacts of participation in a confidential enquiry panel. Regional Maternity Surveys Office/Northern & Yorkshire Public Health Observatory
3. Maternal and Child Health Research Consortium 1995 Part 1: Summary of methods and main results. In: CESDI 2nd annual report. Department of Health, London
4. Northern Regional Health Authority Coordinating Group 1984 Perinatal mortality: a continuing collaborative regional survey. British Medical Journal 288: 1717–1720
5. Confidential Enquiries into Stillbirths and Deaths in Infancy 2003 Project 27/28: an enquiry into quality of care and its effect on the survival of babies born at 27/28 weeks. The Stationery Office, London
6. Hawthorne G, Robson S, Ryall EA, Sen D, Roberts SH, Ward Platt MP 1997 Prospective population based survey of outcome of pregnancy in diabetic women: results of the Northern Diabetic Pregnancy Audit, 1994. British Medical Journal 315: 279–281
7. Hawthorne GC, Wright C 1999 Confidential enquiry as a tool in diabetic pregnancy care. Practical Diabetes International 16: 71–72
8. Maternal and Child Health Consortium 1999 CESDI 6th annual report. Department of Health, London
9. Derrington MC, Gallimore S 1997 The effect of the national confidential enquiry into perioperative deaths on clinical practice. Report of a postal survey of a sample of consultant anaesthetists. Anaesthesia 52: 3–8
10. Foy R, Nelson F, Penney GC 2000 Awareness of key recommendations from the report on confidential enquiries into maternal deaths 1994–96 among obstetric and midwifery staff in Scotland. Journal of Clinical Excellence 2: 27–32
11. National Confidential Enquiry into Perioperative Deaths 2002 Functioning as a team? The 2002 report of the national confidential enquiry into perioperative deaths. NCEPOD, London
12. Ward Platt MP, Brown K, on behalf of the Ashington Evaluation Group. In press. Evaluation of advanced neonatal nurse practitioners: confidential enquiry into the management of sentinel cases. Archives of Disease in Childhood

Chapter **9**

Past, present and future for the confidential enquiries
Richard Congdon

The feelings of grief and distress from mothers and their partners at the death of their babies cannot be overestimated and it is important that the service strives to bring the rate down even further.[1]

WHAT IS A 'NATIONAL CONFIDENTIAL ENQUIRY?'

National confidential enquiry is undoubtedly a highly valuable tool for improving clinical practice, but all the current national enquiries are very different. What do they have in common?

I would suggest four significant common features:

1. Records are anonymized as regards patients, clinicians and healthcare providers.
2. Individual cases are examined in an attempt to learn lessons that can be applied generally.
3. Predetermined standards are used to assess the care provided and the impact on outcomes.
4. It is a peer review process.

The system is about learning not blaming. Practising clinicians are happy to get involved and are willing to identify where clinical practice has failed to live up to expected standards. The enquiries give a no-holds barred snapshot of current practice but they do this in a way which is supported by professionals. Recommendations for improvement are more likely to be accepted by clinicians because the underlying process is one in which they have been fully involved.

The approach has some similarities to clinical audit and has sometimes been described as a form of national clinical audit. The confidential enquiry methodology is beginning to evolve quite rapidly. Confidential enquiries in the future are likely to see a greater amalgamation of audit and research techniques with the aim of producing more scientifically robust findings.

EVOLUTION OF THE CONFIDENTIAL ENQUIRIES

Maternal deaths

Confidential enquiries into maternal deaths started early in the last century in response to variable rates of avoidable maternal mortality in different parts of the country. Initially, these were short term, locally based studies, which then broadened out into time-limited national enquiries. In 1952, the national Confidential Enquiries into Maternal Deaths (CEMD) was set up on an ongoing basis. It enquires into all deaths of mothers from the birth of their baby to 12 months after delivery. The approach is observational and is based on pooling the collective experience and knowledge of regional and national clinical assessors to produce aggregated findings.

It was introduced in response to pressure from clinicians who wanted to find a way in which lessons could be learned from a maternal death for all clinicians involved in maternal care, and to prevent a recurrence wherever possible. The national confidential enquiries have continued to enjoy a strong measure of ownership by clinical professionals. It is very important that this part of their identity is retained.

The maternal enquiry is based on a triennial cycle with a major report covering all the principal causes of deaths. The rate of maternal deaths has fallen dramatically in the last 50 years along with a very substantial change in the causes of those deaths. One of the key findings of the maternal enquiry in recent years has been the enormous importance of social exclusion as a factor in rates of maternal mortality. The most recent report identified that women from the most disadvantaged groups of society were about 20 times more likely to die than women in the highest two social classes.

Perinatal mortality

In 1992 the Confidential Enquiries into Stillbirths and Deaths in Infancy (CESDI) was set up as an ongoing national enquiry. This was in response to concerns that, although the infant mortality rate had fallen each year from 1970, it was levelling out at a higher rate than that found in some other developed countries.

The national enquiry was introduced by instituting a national secretariat to coordinate the efforts of freestanding regional perinatal mortality surveys that had been set up prior to CESDI.

CESDI collected data on late fetal losses from 20 weeks' gestation to 12 months old. A number of major studies were completed by CESDI, including studies into sudden unexpected deaths in infancy and deaths of babies born at 27–28 weeks' gestation.

Other national enquiries

Two other national confidential enquiries have been set up on an ongoing basis; these are the National Confidential Enquiry into Perioperative Deaths (NCEPOD) and the Confidential Inquiry into Suicides and Homicides (CISH).

CURRENT POSITION ON CONFIDENTIAL ENQUIRIES

NICE strategy for national confidential enquiries

In 1999 the National Institute for Clinical Excellence (NICE) took over responsibility for the commissioning of the four national confidential enquiries that were in existence at that time. This has ushered in a period of major change for all the enquiries.

NICE undertook a strategic review with the following main conclusions:

- CEMD and CESDI would be merged to form the Confidential Enquiry into Maternal and Child Health (CEMACH).

- CEMACH would have its terms of reference extended to include the setting up of a new national confidential enquiry into child health.

- Confidential enquiries would be enabled to bring morbidity and near misses within their scope.

- A substantial redistribution of resources would take place between confidential enquiries, so that the opening budget of CEMACH would be some 60% (£1.27 m) of the combined budgets of CESDI and CEMD. The money released would be used to expand the scope of NCEPOD and CISH.

- The methodologies of the enquiries would be developed to include greater scientific rigour. This would include the application of the case-control approach to the enquiry methodology. The importance of denominator data was also identified.

Setting up the confidential enquiry into maternal and child health

CEMACH was set up in April 2003. Although its establishment was a key element in a radical change programme, care has been taken to retain the strengths of CESDI and CEMD as far as possible in setting up CEMACH.

CEMACH has retained a system of regional offices with nine such offices in England matching the government offices for the regions. It has affiliated offices in Northern Ireland and Wales. The regional infrastructure is valuable in enabling the enquiry to maintain local networks, which, in turn, support high levels of ascertainment and the holding of regional multidisciplinary enquiry panels based on the involvement of practising local clinicians. This is a very successful way of ensuring that trusts and clinicians around the country remain actively and positively committed to the enquiry's work.

CEMACH is managed by the professions whose work it evaluates. At the heart of its board is a consortium of royal colleges with members nominated from the following colleges:

- Faculty of Public Health (FPH)
- Royal College of Anaesthetists (RCA)
- Royal College of Midwives (RCM)
- Royal College of Obstetricians and Gynaecologists (RCOG)
- Royal College of Paediatricians and Child Health (RCPCH)
- Royal College of Pathologists (RCPath).

The RCOG hosts the enquiry in the sense that the contract for the provision of the enquiry's services is formally between the RCOG and NICE. However, the RCOG undertakes this responsibility to provide support to the enquiry's work and does not seek any greater influence on the enquiry's work than any other of the colleges on the consortium.

The first chair of CEMACH is Professor Michael Weindling, a neonatologist and member of the RCPCH.

Work programme inherited by the confidential enquiry into maternal and child health

In March 2003, CEMD was at a critical point in its triennial cycle. One 3-year cycle had been completed in December 2002 and a new one had been started in January 2003, which will run until December 2005. It is the intention of CEMACH to complete the reports on these two triennia using the methodology that had applied prior to it taking on the maternal enquiry.

CESDI was engaged in three studies at its dissolution in March 2003:

1. The ongoing collection of perinatal mortality data through the 'rapid report form' (RRF) system.
2. Project 27/28 on outcomes for babies born at between 27 and 28 weeks' gestation.
3. Diabetic pregnancies.

CEMACH will seek to ensure that all these strands of work are recognized within its own work programme. More detail on the plans for integrating this inherited work within the overall programme for CEMACH is given below.

FUTURE PLANS

Confidential enquiries into maternal and child health programme: overview

Initially, the work undertaken by CEMACH will be primarily derived from its two predecessor bodies. This reflects the extensive work-in-progress it has inherited of projects at various stages of completion. The ultimate ambition is that CEMACH will run an enquiry programme that at any point in time has projects drawn from each of the areas for which it has been given responsibility:

- The maternal enquiry (from CEMD)
- The perinatal enquiry (from CESDI)
- A new child health enquiry.

There is no doubt that in some areas of its responsibility CEMACH could beneficially collaborate with NCEPOD or CISH by conducting joint studies. This is something that CEMACH is keen to explore for the future.

It is the clear aim of CEMACH that all areas included in its brief should be constantly on its agenda. To achieve a concurrent programme of enquiries in all three of these areas will not be achieved immediately. The diabetes project is such a major piece of work that in the early days of the new enquiry it will absorb a large part of CEMACH's capacity.

Diabetes project

In the first few months of the new enquiry substantial work has already been committed to establishing the continuity and future direction of the diabetes project, which will represent a major part of the early work programme for CEMACH.

The diabetes project is an important project based on the collection of a dataset of 18 months of diabetic pregnancies in England, Wales and Northern Ireland. Diabetic pregnancies continue to result in a significantly greater rate of stillbirths, infant deaths and congenital malformations than for the population as a whole. On reviewing the position in April 2003, the new enquiry has opted to view the diabetes study as a modular project consisting of four interrelated but distinct phases, which should each result in a published report:

- The diabetes organizational survey – this report will be based on the results of a questionnaire completed by trusts of how periconceptional, antenatal and postnatal services for diabetic women are managed.

- The analysis of the dataset – the dataset collected for the diabetes project contains a unique range and depth of information on diabetic pregnancies and a report will be published analyzing the current position and the issues raised.

- The report of the enquiry – this will set out the results of the reviews undertaken by the enquiry panels of a sample of cases drawn from the dataset with a report on the care provided based on an assessment against recognized standards for the care and treatment of diabetic pregnancy.

- A proposal for a research project – it is intended to prepare a proposal for a research project on important issues raised by the diabetes project. This may focus on standards of periconceptional services and their impact on deaths and malformations.

Perinatal mortality data

CESDI set up a data collection system for the perinatal enquiry. This is the RRF system. It is used to collect data on late fetal losses, stillbirths and deaths in infancy from 20 weeks' gestation to 12 months old. The data collected contains more clinical information than that collected by the Office of National Statistics (ONS).

The system was originally set up to provide an ongoing trend analysis of mortality data for CESDI, as well as cases that could be extracted for sampling for enquiry purposes.

The data have not been directly used for sampling for enquiry cases for some considerable time now, although trend data continue to be provided. The system is also valued by many hospitals for the trend and comparative data it provides. It is, of course, likely that the system will eventually be used again for sampling for enquiry purposes in the future.

CEMACH aims to retain this system, but needs to reduce the resources used in collecting the data to reflect its reduced funding and its increased workload.

The CEMACH strategy for the RRF system has the following main elements:

- Reduced age ranges for which data are collected and the data items collected for each death.
- Development of web-based feedback systems for the hospitals providing the data.
- Development of electronic input of the data.
- Engagement in the national debate about the collection of maternity and birth data as both a collector and user of such data.

The aim will be that CEMACH retains a perinatal mortality data-collection system of value to the national enquiry and to individual hospitals.

Child health

The strategy developed by NICE for the confidential enquiries included the expectation that CEMACH would introduce a new national confidential enquiry into child health. CEMACH is committed to delivering this objective. 'Child' for this purpose is defined as from 28 days to 16 years old. The focus of such studies will not necessarily be confined to deaths, but may also include morbidity and/or disability. The Children's National Service Framework (NSF) is expected to be an important source for this stream of work. The working assumption is that a new child health enquiry will be the first major project to follow the diabetes project.

Maternal enquiry

CEMACH is committed to completing the reports of the maternal enquiry for the triennia ended 31 December 2002 and 31 December 2005 using the same methodology as had been used by CEMD prior to its merger with CESDI and the setting up of the new enquiry.

During 2004 CEMACH will be setting up a review of the maternal enquiry, with a view to introducing any agreed changes to the current system with effect from January 2006. The review will be conducted under the auspices of the CEMACH board and will include significant input from the clinical professions responsible for the care of mothers. It is anticipated that the results of the review will be subject to consultation amongst stakeholders and, following any revisions at consultation stage, will be put to the board and to NICE for final approval.

The maternal enquiry could, in the future, be an area where a joint approach with the other confidential enquiries would be particularly beneficial.

An evolving methodology

There are two key aspects of the methodology for future enquiries to explore in more depth at this stage.

First, there is the central question of the clinical standards to be used as the benchmark for the adequacy of clinical care in enquiries. There are a wide number of bodies recognized as issuing authoritative clinical standards and guidelines for clinicians. Nonetheless, a key responsibility of NICE is the development of national clinical guidelines. Whilst this work has so far attained less public prominence than the technical appraisal of new drugs and therapies, it still represents an essential part of the Institute's work programme.

A central source for future enquiries can, therefore, be expected to be the standards contained in the clinical guidance issued by NICE. CEMACH will, of course, continue at the same time to use clinical standards derived from other sources where this is appropriate.

Second, there is the issue of the application of the case-control approach to the confidential enquiry methodology. The intention is that CEMACH will carry out studies using case controls wherever possible. As a result, the confidential enquiry methodology used by CEMACH is expected to evolve from a form of national clinical audit into a hybrid of clinical audit and research. This process had already started in the design of Project 27/28, which used a case-control approach.

Implications and benefits of using case controls in confidential enquiries

The use of case controls will represent a significant commitment for CEMACH. Greater time and resource will need to be put into project design. The selection of matching cases for control purposes will need care. Sample sizes will be determined primarily by the need to ensure studies with results that achieve high levels of confidence in statistical terms rather than by the capacity of the organization to undertake them. Results will require careful statistical analysis. The enquiry will need to make sure that it has access to high levels of expertise, not only in clinical care and epidemiology, but also in research methodology and statistics.

What benefits are expected to flow from the significant additional commitment implied by using a case-control methodology when compared to a 'simple' clinical audit approach? The first main benefit is that the results of enquiry work should be more scientifically robust. There is a risk with the traditional confidential enquiry approach (i.e. no controls) that substandard clinical practice will be identified and that it will be concluded that it has been a contributory factor in an adverse outcome. However, it is possible that the prevalence of sub-standard clinical practice in relation to a standard is the same where there has been a successful outcome and that it is, therefore, not significant in determining outcomes. Only where a case-control approach is being followed will it be possible to test this. The results should therefore, be significantly more robust (although perhaps less likely to be sensationalist!) where a case-control approach is being followed.

Even so, some caution will still be needed. The events reviewed in confidential enquiries are drawn from real-life cases and are invariably complex. Those events will continue to require interpretation by experienced professionals. There will, therefore, continue to be an important role for informed professional opinion in assessing whether the clinical practice in a case under review met the standards defined as acceptable by the enquiry.

The second main benefit should be in the use to which enquiry findings can be put by NICE as the principal commissioner for the work. Future enquiries should increasingly be able to advise NICE about whether practising clinicians are aware of, and are following, its guidance. Where it is also possible to apply case controls, the results of the enquiry should be able to provide information on whether the application of the standards promulgated by NICE leads to a discern-ible difference in clinical outcomes. Confidential enquiry is, thus, a potentially highly powerful tool for the assessment and review of published clinical guidelines.

SUMMARY AND CONCLUSIONS

CEMACH will develop an enquiry programme that will, at any one time, cover all three areas for which it is responsible, i.e. mothers, babies and children. Over time it will seek to develop consistent methodologies for all areas of its enquiry programme. It will also aim to work collaboratively with the other national confidential enquiries in carrying out specific projects.

Key values and approaches from the past will be retained because they are fundamental to the success of the enquiry process. CEMACH sees itself as rooted in the clinical professions and owned by them – hence, the importance of the consortium of royal colleges on its board. The aim of the enquiry will continue to be to learn from actual cases and to improve clinical practice without attaching blame. Wider issues with a public-health significance will continue to be highlighted. The whole process will retain absolute rigour regarding the confidentiality of the patients, clinicians and hospitals involved in any case.

CEMACH will continue to strive to strengthen the scientific rigour of its findings by ensuring consistency in its approach across the country. It will apply appropriate methodologies, including the case-control approach, wherever possible to ensure that its findings are evidence based. It will aim to strengthen its links with the clinical guideline development programme of NICE by being able to report on the level of implementation of such guidelines across the country, and by assessing their impact on outcomes for patients.

The future for CEMACH looks both demanding and exciting. We hope that clinicians across the country will be fully involved in the study programme as it develops. This will continue to be a fundamental part of the enquiry's identity.

Reference

1. Department of Health 1993 Changing childbirth, part 1. Report of the Expert Maternity Group. HMSO, London

Index

Page numbers in *italics* refer to Figures and Tables.